P

BEFORE, AFDRE, AND A...

"Before, Afdre, and After will break your heart, make you smile, and ultimately make you proud to know people like Maureen Twomey breathe the same air we all do."

—Rob Schwartz, Global Creative President, TBWA\Worldwide

"I never thought I'd say this and mean it: This book will make you laugh and it will make you cry. It's a joyous, inventive journey through loss and recovery, and Maureen's spirit shines through in this blueprint for living a full, blessed and loving life. Read it now, you fools!!"

—Jeff Kreisler, author of *Get Rich Cheating*

"Brave. Wow. Godspeed, Maureen."

—Lee Clow, Director Media Arts, TBWA\ Worldwide, Chairman, Media Arts Lab

BEFORE, AFDRE, and AFTER

(My stroke ...
oh what fun)

MAUREEN TWOMEY
(and Many Other People Too)

Advertising people: You and I think it should be *Before, Afdre and After* (no second comma). But many other people think it should have the second comma. One expert said, "Some people think it looks cluttered. But there are some cases where you really need it."

So I gave in: *Before, Afdre, and After*

Published 2015
Printed in the United States of America
ISBN: 978-0-9863315-0-3
Library of Congress Control Number: 2015903921

For information, address:
Maureen Twomey
maureentwomey.wordpress.com

Cover and interior design by Tabitha Lahr

For my family and
my friends

. . . And a very special
thank you to the team at
Warner Coaching, who
helped me in countless
ways to make this book
a reality

Be safe:

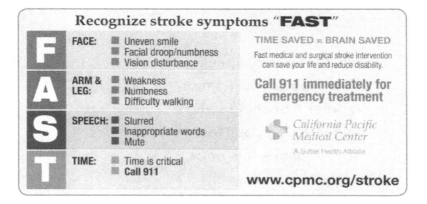

American Stroke Association

www.stroke.org

National Stroke Association

www.stroke.org

www.stroke.org/site/PageServer?pagename=FMD

INTRODUCTION

Hi, I'm Maureen Twomey. When I was only 33, June 6, 2000, I had a stroke. It was HUGE. (??!!)

I didn't expect it. (Well . . . no one *does*.) I was healthy, fit, had low blood sugar, etc. So what happened?

It turns out that I had a rare type of stroke: a "stroke secondary to fibromuscular dysplasia," which usually occurs in young females. Some people who have fibromuscular dysplasia do NOT GET A STROKE. But I did . . . lucky me (rrrrrrr).

The stroke caused a tear in my internal carotid artery.

Stroke secondary to fibromuscular dysplasia: Damage to brain tissue caused by fibromuscular dysplasia, an inherited disorder that leads to the destruction of arterial blood vessels, which can cause bleeding in the brain.

It was June 6, 2000, and I was at work on my computer. And all of a sudden, I was on the floor. "What's happening to me!?" I asked. "Am I having a stroke?" My coworkers didn't know.

Soon the emergency team came and took me to the hospital, where they did a CAT Scan of my brain. But fibromuscular dysplasia is lower (arterial), and they didn't check that low at first. So they told me they were going to do some more tests . . .

They didn't find the stroke until the next day: June 7, 2000.

It's not the hospital's fault whatsoever. It's my ARTERY and my BRAIN'S fault. I would sue, but I can't.

Damn it!

Anyway, I'm doing much better now, but I still have a ways to go . . .

June 22, 2000, I finally understood that I'd had a stroke. My first thought was

"AAAAAAAAAH!"

The second thing I thought was,

"AAAAAAAAAAAAAAAAH!"

Then—not immediately, but after a while—the third thing I thought was: "Hey, I have a GREAT story to tell!"

The problem was, I couldn't tell it. The stroke had taken everything away. I couldn't read or write or even speak. I couldn't tell my story at all . . .

AAAAAAAAAAAAAAAAAAAA AAAAAAAAAAAAAAAAAAAAAH!

"Well hey," I thought, "I'm not a genius, but I am gifted . . ."

> **GIFTED:** *Talented; a special, often creative or artistic, aptitude . . .*

". . . So two weeks from now— three weeks tops—I'll be 100 percent better," I decided. "And soon I will be done with my book. A story about how I did it.

"After all, many people have a stroke or experience a brain injury and lose the ability to read or write . . . but in time, a lot of them recover those abilities," I thought.

Well, I not only had a stroke caused by fibromuscular dysplasia, I also developed dysgraphia AND aphasia AND apraxia AND brain injury AND cognitive deficits.

Hmmmmm . . . Well, maybe it would take longer to write my story than I first thought.

Now, more than a decade later, I am able to read and write and speak much better than I could at first, but I am still not as accomplished at these things as I was before my stroke (not yet, anyway!).

So some people helped me along the way, of course. Ellen Gilbert, MS, my reading, writing, speech, and language teacher, helped me tremendously at first as I worked to re-learn these skills.

When I first got started, I mostly dictated and Ellen typed what I said. Then I got better at writing, so I

> **RE-LEARN:** *to learn again what has been partly or completely forgotten.*

started typing myself. (Franklin and Talk are key . . . More on this later.)

Of course, I'm typing with only ONE hand on the computer now, because my right arm doesn't work anymore. If you wrote a book with only one hand, YOU would be slow too! (Duh.)

Chuck and MaryAnn LaMere, my uncle and aunt, also helped me when I was getting started. ("Chuck, how do you spell . . ." "MaryAnn, how do you spell . . ." "MaryAnn or Chuck, how do you spell . . ." blab, blab, blab . . .)

When you see Jack Twomey's (my dad's) letters to everyone in the following pages, it is truly Jack/Dad who wrote them. And many more people wrote stuff for this memoir, too.

Mostly, though, I wrote this book. Maybe someone else could tell the story of what happened much better than I can. Maybe my writing isn't as good as it was before. But I've accomplished so much that I want to write it—not have someone else do it for me.

So if this book doesn't come CLOSE to that of a great writer like J.D. Salinger or Harper Lee or Anne Lamott, it is ONLY because—well, YOU know.

Anyway, hopefully you'll enjoy this book. I would say, "If not, maybe you can contact the publisher and say you want your money back," but I'm self-publishing . . . so if you don't like my book, maybe just sell it on Amazon or eBay?

;-)

P.S.: By the way: As you can see, I'm writing only on one half of the page. It's not because I want to use some fancy style, but because I can't see on the right. (I lost vision on the right side in both eyes after my stroke.)

When I was fine I could see all the way a cross the page . . .
. . . .
. . . .

Now, as I write this, I am not able to see the right side of this page. Some people who have had a stroke have this difficulty too. So, I have purposely chosen to use this formatting . . .

Well, I CAN physically turn my head to the right and see there is still print so I can read some more. But in order to do that, I have to turn my head

back	and forth
and back	and forth
and back	and forth . . .
It's like a	tennis match.
Back	and forth . . .
Back	and forth . . .
AAAAAAAH!	I can't take it!

I'll make you a deal:

❀ When I am writing about the time before the stroke, I will make the words go entirely across the page.

❀ When I include writing from my dad, the hospital, friends, etc., you'll know that it's not me writing, because it will also go across the page.

❀ But when I'm writing about everything that happened after the stroke, I'll stick to this half-page formatting. It reinforces the idea that now I can't see the right side.

So that means that while this book at first seems really long, it's actually only 40 pages total.

(Well, maybe a bit more.)

P.P.S.: Of course, as you can see, I'm writing both on the left and right side of this book. It would be over the top to have the entire page on the right side blank. All so, it's saving some paper too.

BEFORE

:)

(CHAPTER 1)

Checklist:

June 5, 2000 and Before:

Read:	☑ Yes
Write:	☑ Yes
Speak:	☑ Yes
Walk:	☑ Yes
Run:	☑ Yes
Drive:	☑ Yes
Good sense of humor:	☑ Yes (?)

I was born in a hospital in Santa Clara, California, and . . . oh, wait a minute; maybe you couldn't care less where I was born. Moving forward . . . eighteen years later I went to UCLA, where I majored in communication and had a great time. I stayed in Los Angeles after college and worked for a creative advertising firm. Do you want to see my resume?

"Yes, Maureen."

Okay. Resume:

Maureen Twomey
Santa Monica, CA 90404

310-

WRITING EXPERIENCE	**TBWA/Chiat/Day, Venice/Playa del Rey** *Copywriter (6/96 - Present)* Nissan, The Weather Channel, ABC, Infiniti, BizRate.com, Samsonite, The Entertainment Industry Foundation, New Business.

MCA Records, Universal City
Editor and Chief Writer, AMP (MCA Records On Line) (4/96 - 7/96)
My issues 8, 9 and 10 were on archive at www.mcarecords.com. Now the archives
are gone and all you can find is really bad/trying-too-hard-to-be-hip writing. Yikes.

Ketchum Advertising, Los Angeles
Copywriter (5/94 - 4/96)
Acura automobiles, PacifiCare, KFC Co-op, Aid For AIDS, New Business.

OTHER
EXPERIENCE

Traffic Coordinator/Traffic Forwarder (2/93 - 5/94)
Acura automobiles, American Lung Association.

Bozell Advertising, Los Angeles
Account Group Assistant; Interoffice Coordinator (10/91 - 2/93)
Rockwell International, Kawasaki Motors Corp., Childhelp U.S.A.

Rubin Postaer & Associates, Los Angeles
Account Group Secretary (11/90 - 9/91) – Honda automobiles.

EDUCATION

WSAAA Creative Course (formerly the Carson Roberts Creative Course)
November, 1994 - April, 1995.

The Bookshop
January - November, 1992.

University of California, Los Angeles
B.A. Communication Studies - June, 1990.

AWARDS
AND HONORS

- 1998 Clios (finalist)
- 1997 *Communication Arts* Advertising Annual
- 1997 New York Art Directors (finalist)
- 1997 and 1996 Beldings
- 1997 One Show (Well, not yet a pencil, but they did display my work in their "Cross Dressing: The Role of Design in Advertising" exhibit – which is even more of an honor, considering I'm not a transvestite.)
- 1995 Best of Ketchum
- 1994 and 1993 Los Angeles Creative Club Student Competition

(Can you tell what is wrong with this? I should have said "TBWA\Chiat\Day," not "TBWA/Chiat/Day." Sorry, TBWA\Chiat\Day. And yes, I covered up my address and phone number, in case you were wondering.)

Anyway, I was thirty-two years young and I was working as a copywriter in advertising. Was I a good one? Well, people at least thought I had a quirky (i.e., good) sense of humor.

I was working for TBWA\Chiat\Day (in L.A.). I got to work on Nissan, Infiniti, The Weather Channel, some ABC ads, The Entertainment Industry Foundation, etc. I did ads for BizRate.com and Samsonite (really humorous baggage claim posters) when we were pitching for those accounts, too, but I can't remember now if I ever got to work on them when we got them . . . hmmm. Well, regardless, it was a great place to work: very creative ads and good people. Also, they had fantastic parties.

I liked doing print ads, but I wanted to do more TV ads, and I wasn't getting a lot of those (only one spot for Nissan and one spot for The Entertainment Industry Foundation). So in November 1999, I said good-bye to TBWA\Chiat\Day and started freelancing for another firm. And I liked it . . . but I still wasn't doing TV. Maybe soon?

In late November, one of my headhunters, Marc Deschenes, told me that another firm in San Francisco—Goldberg Moser O'Neill (GMO)—wanted to see me. I thought it was freelancing only, but it was a full-time job.

I had just started freelancing; maybe I liked that better, I told Marc. But he told me that my former boss from TBWA\Chiat\Day, John Avery, was now working at GMO, and it was a good firm. "Just see the place and talk to them," he said.

I called GMO, and they said they would fly me up and introduce me to the firm. I agreed to come and take a look.

Soon after, I heard that Kia (the car company) was parting ways with GMO:

> *November 18, 1999: "Kia Motors America said Wednesday it has fired San Francisco's Goldberg Moser O'Neill as its advertising agency—a surprise move just weeks after the car maker publicly praised GMO for helping raise its public profile with an ongoing series of humorous ads . . ."*
>
> —(John O'Dell, *Los Angeles Times*)

??!!!

I called John Avery immediately. "Should I not come?" I asked him.

"No, come up still," John said. "The head of Creative said there are many other accounts; not to worry."

So I went up there . . . and I liked them! They had a good sense of humor and a number of great accounts, including Cisco Systems, MicronPC.com, Lucas Art Entertainment, Monterey Bay Aquarium, Audible.com, inTune Hearing Center Solutions, and more.

So I accepted the job, hoping that I would get more TV ads there. I would move up and start my job on January 6, 2000.

I moved to San Francisco to work for Goldberg Moser O'Neill in 2000 (I already told you that a paragraph ago—just checking if you're really paying attention). I found a wonderful apartment right away. I could see the whole San Francisco Golden Gate Bridge from my windows. Whoohoooo! I knew where I'd be on the 4th of July.

My apartment and the Golden Gate Bridge:

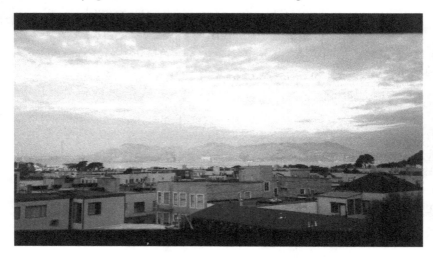

Farther back, you can see Salinger in the picture too:

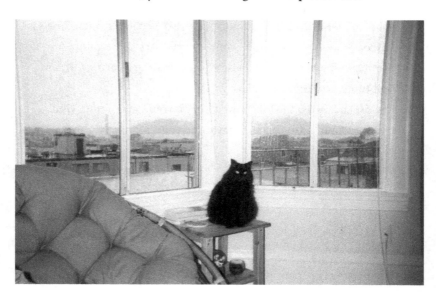

John Neitzel and me at work:

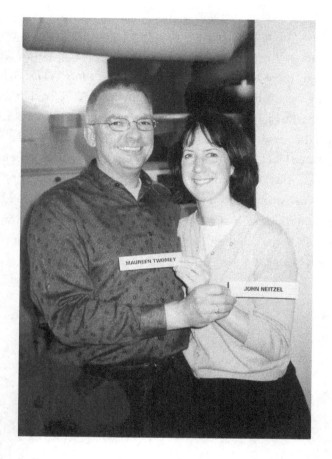

On my first day of work, I had to fill out a number of forms in HR. One form asked how much health insurance coverage I wanted. I was so healthy and fit that at first I thought, "I don't have to get the full coverage. I don't need it." But then I thought, "Hmmm . . . but I'm making more money now, so I can afford it. Well, JUST in case, I will get the full coverage."

(Hey wait, maybe if I hadn't gotten the full insurance, I wouldn't have had a stroke. Shoot . . . Yes, I'm just kidding.)

In L.A., you mostly have to drive; there aren't many buses that will get you anywhere close to where you want to go. In S.F. though, there are TONS of ways to get around WITHOUT taking a car, whether it's buses or Muni or BART. I lived in the Marina/Russian Hill area, and there was a bus stop half a block away. I could take the bus downtown, get off, and only have to walk one block to get to my work! Even better, when you get on the bus, you can read a book at the same time as you're "driving"!

After work, when it wasn't raining or when I didn't have to be somewhere soon, I walked home. There were so many ways to walk home: through Nob Hill, the Tenderloin, Chinatown, North Beach, Russian Hill, and the Marina:

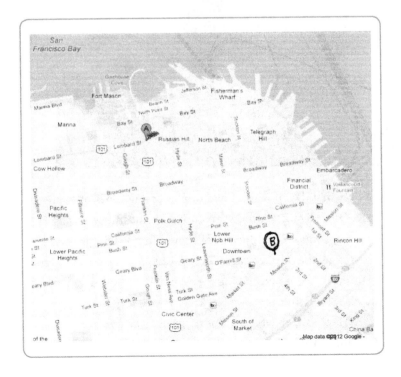

(I think Google is saying right now, "Hey! Why is this map kind of blurry?!" I apologize Google, your maps are always clear. But I had to print it out, scan it, it's now black & white not color etc., so it's not crystal clear in this book.) Here is the real Google maps: https://www.google.com/maps ☺

My work was one block away from Union Square, and three blocks away from the cable cars.

In January (maybe two weeks later), I had a dream:

I was under the water. I was stuck under a rock, so I couldn't get myself up to the surface. I couldn't breathe. I was drowning, and I couldn't do anything about it. I was dying.

Then, suddenly, I could BREATHE, even though I was still UNDERWATER! It was amazing! I realized that I was almost going to heaven . . . but suddenly, I woke up. It was only a dream, and yet it was so real . . .

???

Weird . . .

On January 29, 2000, I went to see Anne Lamott, the author of *Bird by Bird*. The subhead, "Some Instructions on Writing and Life."

Anne Lamott said, "The secret of good writing: bad writing."

"Haaaa!" we laughed.

She explained further, "Really, bad writing means the worst

is over (blank paper). You need something there to work with to end up with 'good writing.'"

"When you're going along the way, write yourself notes about where you might go next," she said. "And remember, if you all of a sudden get an idea, you have to write it all down right away. If you don't write it down now, you'll forget about it."

"She is so right," I thought.

She quoted the author E.L Doctorow: "Writing is like driving at night in the fog. You can only see as far as your headlights, but you can make the whole trip that way."

"What kind of writing do you gravitate toward reading? That's probably what you should be writing," Anne Lamott said.

"There so many things I could write about. So what should I write about first?" I thought. "Hmmmmm . . . I'll think about it some more."

Some friends and I went to watch the BATS Improv comedy show in San Francisco. It was so funny. Here's the website: http://www.improv.org. (But when you get done looking at it, don't forget to come back and continue to read THIS book.)

BATS Improv had classes, too: "All our new students will begin here," their website read, "whether they're interested in becoming improv performers or just want to enjoy learning the skills used in improvisation." Whoohooo!

On February 2, 2000, I went to my first BATS Improv class, a six-week course that they billed as a "fun introduction to the joys and thrills of improvisation and the BATS Improv style."

That class was sooooooo fun.

On March 22, 2000, I turned thirty-three.

... If you still want to give me a present, let me know!

In April of 2000, I took a second six-week BATS class: "Continue the exploration of improvisation while refining improv knowledge and skills . . ."

Another great class.

I began to feel like I wanted to volunteer for something—to give something back to other people who were not as healthy as me. So in May of 2000, I signed up for a breast cancer walk that would be taking place on July 31: a three-day, sixty-mile event.

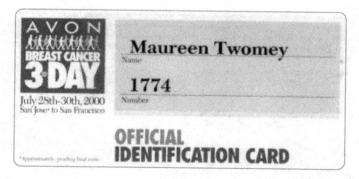

(I think since I had a stroke they should retire the number "1774" as a tribute to me. Mmmmmm Avon?)

Dear friends,

This July 28th – 30th, I'll be walking 60 miles from San Jose to San Francisco for the Avon Breast Cancer 3-Day walk to raise money for breast cancer research and treatment.

Why will I be doing this? Sure, I'm big into walking (mostly because I hate running) but walking 60 miles over three days and camping out with 2000+ others each night is not exactly my idea of a fantastic time. However, besides wanting to help raise money for a great cause, I also have a very personal reason for signing up for the walk.

One day towards the end of my senior year in college, I was extremely alarmed to discover a distinct lump in my breast. At first I didn't tell anyone, because I was far too frightened by the possibility of having it checked and it turning out to be malignant. A couple of weeks later my brain won out over my emotions and I went in to Student Health. They told me that odds were, at my young age, the tumor wasn't cancerous, but that it should still be biopsied. Three days later they operated to remove the tumor. And five days later, I was overwhelmingly relieved to hear that it had indeed been benign.

While my experience with breast cancer was just a scare, **breast cancer is the second leading cause of cancer death for all women, and the leading cause of death in women between the ages of 40 and 55. Plus, one million women in the U.S. currently have breast cancer but don't know it.** And statistically, they won't be diagnosed for another 5-8 years. But even if every one of those women was to be screened and diagnosed today, the cure for and the cause of breast cancer have yet to be discovered.

So I've agreed to raise $2500 in pledges for the Avon Walk by June 30th. This money will help fund non-profit breast health programs in the U.S. and cutting-edge medical research on women's diseases. And as you've guessed by now, I'm writing to ask for your help.

Would you please consider making a pledge to help me meet my $2500 goal? It's fully tax deductible, of course. I've enclosed a pledge form, so if you'd like to make a pledge, please fill it out and send it to the address noted on the form. And if you'd like, I can also send you more details about where the money that's raised will be spent.

Thank you so much in advance. From personal experience, I know that any amount you give to help fund detection programs, treatments and a cure for breast cancer will mean the world to so many.

Sincerely,

Maureen

P.S. Please excuse the "form letter" format! ☺

Man, I think this letter is longer than this book.

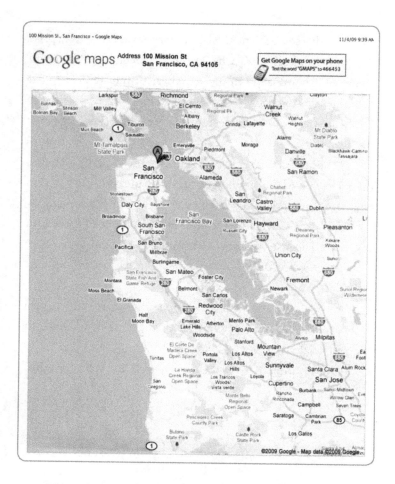

Google maps Address 100 Mission St
San Francisco, CA 94105

Get Google Maps on your phone
Text the word "GMAPS" to 466453

©2009 Google - Map data ©2009 Google

The walk started in San Jose and ended in San Francisco.

Still training for the walk and with several other things I had to do, I went down to L.A. for the weekend, from Friday, June 2 to Sunday, June 4, where I stayed with my friend Stu Gibbs and saw many, many friends.

Saturday some friends, Jill and Mark Savage, had a surprise party for Jenn Muranaka-Chaney (an art director I worked with at TBWA\Chiat\Day). On my way there, I went to 7-11 to get some beer for the party. When I walked in, I walked over to the clerk (he was around nineteen or twenty) and asked, "Where's the beer section?"

He hesitated, but then he said, "Over there" and pointed to the other end of the store. I got the beer, and as I was going to check out the clerk said—totally seriously—"I need some ID."

OH MY GOSH! I had to take my wallet out to show him my driver's license, and now I was smiling.

As soon as I did, the guy said, "Oh, now I can see your wrinkles."

"Hey!" I said, my smile disappearing. "You didn't have to say it out loud!" (Next time I'm buying beer, I'll have to remember: don't smile.)

Anyway, when I got to the party, we all had a terrific time.

☺

(Chapter 2)

Back to San Francisco, Monday, June 5, 2000:

I was fine on Monday, and did my daily routine at work. After work, Bridget, a friend of mine at work, and another guy and I went to the Fillmore to see Elliot Smith (looooooove Elliot Smith). Aaahhhhh . . .

Tuesday, June 6, 2000:

Hey! It's been six months at my job . . . Where's my cake? ;)

It was busy at work, but I left midday for a dermatology appointment. I arrived fifteen minutes early for a 1:30 p.m. appointment.

It was the first time I'd been there, so they'd asked me to come early to fill out some forms. Thankfully, I was going to be the first person of the afternoon to see the dermatologist, which, I thought, meant it would be quick. I waited . . . . 1:30 p.m . . . . 1:45 p.m. . . . 1:55 p.m. . . . 2:00 p.m. . . . "AAAAAAAH!" I thought. "Where's the doctor!? Is she still at lunch? Is she napping?"

FINALLY the doctor showed up. "I have to go back to work!" I said.

She said calmly that she could look me over in five minutes. "Fine!!!" I said.

Suddenly I felt funny, lightheaded, and I wondered what was wrong with me. My right eye was flashing, kind of like a camera: on and off; on and off; on and off. But fifteen seconds later, I felt fine.

Afterward, when I was walking back to work, I was almost crying. "Okay," I told myself, "think about something funny!" (I can't remember what I thought of, but it worked.)

When I got back to work, however, I started to cry.

Later, three women from work—Amy C., Noreen D., and Heather Buhler Jennings—typed a letter saying what they felt had happened to me. They gave it to my dad in the hopes that it could help.

3:00 p.m.

Amy sees Maureen Twomey crying in the hallway in front of Maureen's office. Maureen tells her she has just returned from the dermatologist's office and that her doctor mentioned to her that one side of her is flushed. Maureen is anxious because she is also experiencing flashes of light in one eye and a tingling sensation on one side of her body. She has a slight headache. Amy recommends she call her doctor. Maureen calls and he asks if she's experiencing any pain, to which she replies no. He told her to call back if the headache or other symptoms worsen. Maureen calms herself and continues to work.

4:20 p.m.

Maureen comes into Heather Buhler's office to get cab vouchers from her to go home. One side of her face is droopy, her eyes are crossing, and she is very pale. She says that she has been experiencing flashes of bright light and feels very dizzy and is worried that she might faint. Heather tells her to take a seat and offers her some water. Maureen sits down and begins tearing up; she looks as if she's beginning to panic. Heather asks Maureen to call her doctor and make an appointment and describe her symptoms. Heather goes downstairs to get Maureen cab slips, one to get her to the doctor's office, one to get her home.

I called the doctor again. I had a serious headache. "Maybe it's a migraine?" I thought.

I was thinking, "Tonight was supposed to be my last class of intermediate improv, but I'm so . . . so . . . I don't know what . . . and I have to go home and rest. I have to miss improv even though I don't want to."

4:30 p.m.

Heather returns to Maureen's desk with some cab slips and asks her what her doctor had to say. Maureen says that she is probably suffering from a migraine headache, dehydration, or exhaustion. Maureen wants to go home, so Heather gives Maureen cab slips and asks her to page her if she begins to feel worse. Maureen calls for a cab and begins typing an e-mail to her theatre class notifying them that she will not be in class that evening.

I had to e-mail my improv group to tell them that I would not be there that night. I was on the computer, and then, all of a sudden, I was looking at the words but they didn't make sense to me anymore. It was like they were in a foreign language . . .

(I realized that I could NOT read them now that they looked like, "Eeeeeeeeeeeeeeeeeeeeeee wsoy adwjdke rtyh!?" But I want to tell you more about my story, so I'll still make everything in English . . . okay? Okay.)

. . . and the next second I fell on the floor.
"Oh God . . . What's happening to me?"

4:40 p.m.

Amy, in the next office, hears Maureen fall out of her chair and begin crying. Amy runs into her office and finds her on her back with her head propped up against a filing cabinet. Maureen is holding her head and crying. She is quite frightened and is experiencing a severe headache, the flashes in one eye, and numbness in one arm. Amy asks Noreen to get a cab slip for Maureen to go to the hospital and then calls Maureen's doctor, who tells her to call 911 immediately. They tell her to give the paramedics Maureen's insurance card so the hospital will contact the doctor once she is admitted. One of Maureen's eyes looks droopy. Maureen, still crying, asks Amy if she thinks she's having a stroke.

Amy sits with her, holds her hand, and tries to keep her comfortable and calm until the paramedics arrive just a few minutes later. Several coworkers come to see if they can help in any way. Maureen says she's thirsty. Gloria T. gets Maureen some water, but Maureen says she can't/doesn't want to drink, despite her thirst.

Physically I was wondering, "What does that mean? Maybe if I explain myself they could do something about it more quickly." Again, I thought I was having a stroke . . . But a split second later, I completely forgot about not being able to read the words. I had other things to worry about.

4:45 p.m.

Maureen tells Amy of the e-mail she was typing and asks her to delete it because she was unable to finish it. Amy notices that Maureen had been typing just one letter for a couple of lines towards the end of the note. Noreen and Amy and Gloria sit with Maureen and wait for the paramedics. Amy asks if there's a friend or relative she can call and Maureen dictates her father's phone number to Noreen (Jack Twomey) from memory. Noreen calls and speaks to Maureen's stepmother, Judy Twomey, to tell her she'll be accompanying Maureen to California Pacific. She gives her cell phone number to keep her posted until Mr. Twomey can get to the hospital.

Someone said, "I'm not sure what caused it, but I am sure everything will be all right."

4:50 p.m.

Maureen is able to express herself well, though she mentions that she's having difficulty doing so.

Approximately 4 Fire Department paramedics arrive. They arrive in a fire truck. Maureen is alert and awake. They ask who's in charge and Gloria calls Kathleen J. in HR, who brings up Maureen's health/emergency contact file. Maureen describes to the paramedics her complete history of the day. Her story includes complaints of bright flashes of light behind her eyes, numbness on one side of her body, an inability to type the end of a sentence on her keyboard, and a now severe headache. Maureen IS awake and alert. She asks that someone call her acting class to tell them she can't make it and asks Amy to pack up some work for her to take home.

(What was I thinking?!)

(Amy tells her not to worry about the work.) Maureen is crying and scared. One side of her face is visibly drooping and one side of her face is still flushed. Approximately 3 additional paramedics arrive in an ambulance. The new paramedics interview Maureen and she tells them the same history of her day. Maureen is still crying and frightened but seems to be calmed slightly by the arrival of the paramedics. Different paramedics ask Maureen and Amy questions and take Maureen vitals. At one point they have her standing up, with one paramedic steadying her on each side.

5:00 p.m.

Although there are approximately 7 paramedics at Maureen's desk with her, only two are interviewing her. There is a general feeling among the group that this is not an emergency situation. Some of the paramedics hold separate personal conversations and wait until the two finish their check-up interview. The paramedics who interviewed Maureen listen to her heartbeat while she is lying down, help her stand and take her heartbeat while she's standing, examine her eyes, and conduct a few other routine tests.

The medics put me on a slanted board. I thought I felt better. They then rolled in a gurney that folded into an upright position and took me down to the ambulance in the elevator. I began feeling slightly better but was still visibly shaken.

VERY IMPORTANT SIDE NOTE: THE TIME FACTOR

A stroke is considered an emergency because of the time factor involved. A clot-busting drug called tissue plasminogen activator (tPA) can reduce the amount of permanent damage from a stroke, according to the American Heart Association, but tPA must be administered within three hours of the onset of symptoms to be effective.

Three hours for me on June 6, 2000 was:

2:05 p.m. (When I was in the dermatology office) to 5:05 p.m. (When I was still at work) ☹

... BUT the newer guidelines for tPA recommend use for up to **4.5 hours after the onset of symptoms,** not three hours, though other strict criteria also must be met BEFORE the medicine can be given:

> "Tissue plasminogen activator can be used to treat some people who are having a stroke caused by a blood clot (ischemic stroke) It is given in a vein (intravenously, or IV) and in some cases may be given directly into an artery."

So if I could take it, I should have until 6:35 p.m.! (Of course, I didn't know what tPA was. But thankfully the doctors do know this. If it was a stroke, hopefully I could take tPA!)

5:10 p.m.
The paramedics take Maureen out of the building in the gurney.

As they were bringing me out of the building, I knew I was going to the hospital, but right across the street was a bar/snacks place, and I wanted to go there instead. "Well," I thought, "maybe I will feel better later, and I'll go with my friends then. I will ask the paramedics and fire people if they want to come too, and I can treat them to drinks."

(!?)

Noreen goes with the 3 paramedics and Maureen in the ambulance. Once inside the ambulance, the three paramedics are in back with Maureen and Noreen is sitting in front alone. The fire truck with the other 4 paramedics leaves. One paramedic takes blood samples from Maureen. He also does other tests that Noreen is not closely watching. After approximately 10 minutes inside the ambulance outside of GMO, the third paramedic gets out of the back and gets into the driver seat. The ambulance lights and siren are not on. Ambulance drives through rush hour traffic to get to California Pacific Hospital at Webster and Sacramento. The trip takes approximately 20 minutes. There is not a feeling of emergency within the ambulance. Maureen is heard talking again about her symptoms to a paramedic. Noreen asks Maureen if she can go into Maureen's wallet for her insurance card. Maureen makes a joke about going through her wallet.

5:45 p.m.

Ambulance arrives at hospital. Maureen is admitted on the emergency vehicle's gurney. All three paramedics and Noreen accompany Maureen inside. The paramedics relay the information that they gathered from Maureen to the admitting nurse at the hospital. Maureen also gives the same information to the nurse about the history of her day and her symptoms.

5:50 p.m.

Maureen is put into bed in a shared room (4 beds). Maureen and Noreen are alone for a few minutes and Maureen cries. Maureen speaks again about her symptoms from the day.

5:55 p.m.

The emergency room doctor talks to Maureen about her symptoms for 5 minutes. During Maureen's account of her symptoms, she is distracted by the man in the next bed. There is a drape separating them, but he is grunting and groaning and Maureen tells the doctor that she can't concentrate while he is making the noises . . .

(He was so drunk and farting all the time . . . Aaaaaaaah!)

They finish their conversation and the doctor leaves.

6:05 p.m.

Maureen is annoyed and distressed by the man next to her and asks Noreen to find out if she can be moved.

6:15 p.m.

Maureen is taken upstairs for a CAT Scan. Maureen and Noreen wait in the hallway for the CAT Scan and Noreen asks if Maureen is okay with the Scan. Maureen responds that she had one approximately 6 years previously when she was hit by a car . . .

In 1994, I was crossing the street on the way to work (the arrow was white not red) when a car hit me (she was driving about 5 or 10 miles a hour) and I flew onto the hood and then onto the street. (AAAAAAAH!) Thankfully, she stopped and got out of her car to help me, and an ambulance came right away and took me to the hospital. When I was in the ambulance I just kept saying something like, "Please help me, Lord . . ."

Much later, after the stroke—I think in 2008—I asked Dr. Kitt (M.D., Neurology) if my stroke had anything to do with the car accident. He said it had nothing to do with it.

> . . . Maureen is still in a general nervous and scared state, although not necessarily related to the CAT Scan.

6:20 p.m.
Maureen is CAT Scanned.

Hey, my head is fine . . . No sign of stroke here! Whoohoo!
   (Yeah, right . . .) :-1

6:30 p.m.
Maureen is taken back down to the emergency room, where she is placed in the hallway. She has requested that she not be put in the same bed (next to the man), and there is no other space in the ER. Maureen rests with her eyes shut on her gurney in the hallway.

VERY IMPORTANT SIDE NOTE AGAIN:
2:05 p.m. to 6:35 p.m. . . . . "I still have time left to get the tPA!"

6:36 p.m. → ☹

6:45 p.m.
Noreen talks to Maureen's father on the phone and he leaves for the hospital.

7:15 p.m.

Mr. Twomey arrives at the hospital. The doctor informs Maureen that the CAT Scan showed no evidence of stroke and that they wanted to perform a spinal tap (lumbar puncture) to get a better analysis of her condition. Maureen is very upset by the news of the spinal tap. The doctor reassures Maureen that the test is not painful, but Maureen is still upset and cries. The nurse gives Maureen a drug to relax.

7:30 p.m.

Maureen's drug is starting to work and she is getting groggy. Maureen speaks with her dad briefly about her condition, and then she tells him that she is too tired to talk. Maureen rests with her eyes closed as her father talks.

7:40 p.m.

Maureen and Mr. Twomey are taken into a semi-private room (one other bed) and Maureen seems to be sleeping.

Since there were no more test being done that night, I went to Dad and Judy's house (only fifteen minutes away). Thank heavens I did; if I had gone home—I don't think I would be alive right now.

Judy noticed something funny (well, not funny—strange). I was slurring my words. My right side was drooping. Well, maybe I was just tired. I immediately went to sleep. Having dreams . . . or nightmares . . .

June 7, 2000:

Wednesday, in the morning, I felt the same—so weird. I ate two or three bites of cereal, and I felt SOOOO strange. I had to go back to bed.

Then: "WHAT'S HAPPENING TO ME!!!"

(After this I don't remember much, but I'll tell what I can.)

Dad carried me to the car (he didn't wait for the paramedics to arrive). He put me in the back, so I could lie down, and buckled the seat belt, and then he drove as fast as he could to the emergency room at California Pacific Hospital again.

When we got there, I could not walk at all now. And finally, I could not talk at all.

Blackout.

AFDRE

:(

(Chapter 3)

Checklist:

← June 5, 2000 and Before:

~~Read:~~ ☑ ~~Yes~~

~~Write:~~ ☑ ~~Yes~~

~~Speak:~~ ☑ ~~Yes~~

~~Walk:~~ ☑ ~~Yes~~

~~Run:~~ ☑ ~~Yes~~

~~Drive:~~ ☑ ~~Yes~~

~~Good sense of humor:~~ ☑ ~~Yes (?)~~

Afdre → Jd?! 6~@ 2#%! | (After → June 6/7, 2000)

Afdre → Jd?! 6~@ 2#%!		(After → June 6/7, 2000)	
Rehc:	☹	(Read:	☒ No)
Wy5vy:	☹	(Write:	☒ No)
Srvjy:	☹	(Speak:	☒ No)
Whnl:	☹	(Walk:	☒ No)
Rjc:	☹	(Run:	☒ No)
Dtwxg:	☹	(Drive:	☒ No)
Gqau srube qb enuie:	☹	(Good sense of humor:	☒ No)

CALIFORNIA PACIFIC MEDICAL CENTER

TWOMEY, MAUREEN   ADMIT: 06/07/00
INTERIM SUMMARY

HISTORY OF PRESENT ILLNESS: The patient is a 33-year-old female who was brought in by her father for right-sided weakness. The patient had been seen in the emergency department the day prior with symptoms of headache with some flashing light symptoms in both eyes. At that time the patient denied any numbness or weakness. She had a possible history of migraines. The patient did have a head CT scan which was negative. She also underwent a lumbar puncture which showed a normal cell count, protein and glucose. The patient remained in the emergency room a while longer and was able to be discharged home. Upon waking up on the morning of admission the patient's father noted her to have unusual speech with difficulty expressing herself. She also had a headache. At that time he also note right arm weakness. The patient stayed in bed for several hours further, and then when she tried to get out of bed she fell. The patient has no prior history of neurologic symptoms in the past except for possible migraines. She has no history of stroke, or hypercoagulable state.

PAST MEDICAL HISTORY: None, according to the father.

(Phillip Kennedy, M.D.)

Many Doctors:

Dr. Donald Kitt, M.D., Neurology

Dr. Brian Andrews, M.D., Neurology Surgery

Dr. Lawrence Goldyn, M.D., Internal Medicine

Dr. Phillip Kennedy, M.D., Internal Medicine

Dr. Jeremy Berge, M.D., Internal Medicine

Dr. Peter Weber, M.D., Neurology Surgery

Dr. Lory Wiviott, M.D., Internal Medicine

Dr. Fabiola Cobarrubias, M.D., Internal Medicine

Dr. Scott Rome, M.D., Physical Medicine, Rehabilitation

(Davies Campus)

And many more . . . Wow, I guess I'm popular.

(I was still unconscious, so other people told me what they saw after.)

A nurse asked my dad, "Do you think she was in a fight?" (My head was swollen now.)

He said, "She doesn't fight at all. It's not an accident or a fight that did that . . ."

I think it was in the evening that they found the problem. Donald Kitt, M.D. (Neurolgy) wrote:

" . . . She was noted to have a right hemiplegia and a CT scan was done. This study was reviewed to show evolution of an area of acute infarction in the left occipital temporal and poster parietal lobe with loss of the insular ribbon and a hyperdense left MCA sign. This finding was consistent with a left middle cerebral and posterior cerebral acute in-

farction. Fetal circulation of the left
PCA was postulated . . ."

> **EVOLUTION:** the gradual development of something, esp. from a simple to a more complex form; advancement, growth, rise, progress, expansion . . .
>
> **ACUTE:** (of a bad, difficult, or unwelcome situation or phenomenon) present or experienced to a severe or intense degree . . .
>
> **INFARCTION:** the obstruction of the blood supply to an organ or region of tissue, typically by a thrombus or embolus, causing local death of the tissue.

So finally, the doctors diagnosed it:
it was a rare form of stroke.

> **Stroke secondary to fibromuscular dysplasia (again):** Damage to brain tissue caused by fibromuscular dysplasia, an inherited disorder that leads to the destruction of arterial blood vessels, which can cause bleeding in the brain.

I guess they didn't see it the first day because it was small. But my head was now swollen, so they saw the stroke.

Dr. Andrews, the head of the Neurology Surgery team, told my family that there was so much swelling they had to temporarily remove a part of my skull or I would die. He'd had only one other case like this before, he said, and it was a motorcycle accident.

Bill Twomey (my uncle) was walking up and down the hallway praying: "God! We need a miracle and we need it NOW. Are you listening to me Lord!?"

Thursday, when the surgery was done, Dr. Andrews thought that I was getting better.

Friday morning, Dad went to get my car at my apartment. William Johnson (my next-door neighbor) agreed to take care of my cat, Salinger.

While Dad was gone, I took a turn for the worse. Dr. Andrews told the family that there was still too much swelling . . .

In a letter Dad wrote on June 14, 2000:

On Friday, even though the operation on Thursday was considered successful, there was a sudden increase in the inter-cranial pressure on the brain stem, which is "control central" for the brain. To relieve this pressure, the doctors had to go back in through the opening they had created on Thursday, and remove some of the damaged brain tissue in the left temporal lobe . . .

My brothers, Mike and Kevin, and my cousin, Terri, were there, but Dad was not. And they couldn't make the decision. Terri said to the doctor, "If you had a daughter and she had the same thing as Maureen has, what would YOU do?"

He said, "No question, I would do the surgery."

Dad came back right then, and he said, "Do the surgery."

Dr. Andrews returned after and said, "We've done the surgery. She's still alive. Now all we can do is hope."

My family and the GMO people knew what was going on with me; soon other people knew, too.

Then Joan Twomey (my sister in-law) had saved a bunch of my previous e-mails, and she looked at all the e-mail forwarding addresses listed at the top of my e-mails and wrote to those people about my stroke.

I was back in bed, but I was still unconscious (well, DUH). A nurse came in to change my nightgown. When the nightgown came up my waist, still unconscious, I pulled my gown down—maybe because I was shy?

Dad was there, and after he got home he said to the family something like, "Good to know that Maureen is still lady-like."

Seven days later—Tuesday, June 14, 2000—I woke up. I thought I was in a dream. It was so, SO weird. I felt like I was on drugs. Well, I WAS on drugs, just not illegal drugs. I didn't remember the stroke . . . yet . . .

June 14, 2000
Dear friends of Maureen,

You have already heard that Maureen has suffered a stroke. For those of you who know only a few details, I would like to expand on that and bring you up to date on her current condition. I am Maureen's father, Jack Twomey.

Maureen was at work (Goldberg Moser O'Neill) a week ago Tuesday, June 6. At some time in the afternoon, she complained about a headache, feeling bad. Eventually she fell off of her chair. One of her coworkers, Noreen Doherty, took her to the Emergency Room at California Pacific Medical Center. Over Tuesday and Wednesday, it became evident that Maureen had suffered a stroke and that it was massive. The common types of strokes are infarctions—having to do with blood clots—and "bleeds." Maureen's stroke is of a very unusual type called a "dissection of the carotid artery." In her case, the left carotid artery; that is the one just to the left of your Adam's apple, if you have one. The artery has an outer wall and an inner wall, just like a inner tube in a tire. A tear occurred in the inner wall and blood flowed out into the space between the inner and outer walls. The blood flowing into this space encountered resistance and began collapsing the inner wall of the artery, eventually closing it off. This cut off blood to the forward two-thirds of her left brain.

There was a complication that Maureen has had from the time she was a fetus. In most people, there is a "Y" in the carotid artery, with the main part of the "Y" feeding the forward two-thirds of the brain and the other part of the "Y" going toward the back of the brain. Both sides have this setup. Usually this secondary part of the "Y" is small and does not do a lot of work. In Maureen's case, it is larger and has done quite a bit of the work in supplying blood for the rear one-third of her brain. Thus, when the carotid artery was shut off, there was damage to a portion of the rear one-third, again on her left side.

So there are a lot of bad things that have happened to her, but there are also some good things, especially in the last few days.

First of all, it is a massive stroke and Maureen has lost a lot of brain function. The damage is permanent and irreversible. She is paralyzed on her right side. She has lost vision on the right side in both eyes. She has lost her ability to communicate, both orally and in writing. That is the bad part.

On the good side, first of all, she is alive. During the last week she was in real danger of not making it. But she has.

The biggest problem was her intracranial (blood) pressure. It had to be kept within acceptable limits. The doctors have won this battle. On Thursday, she had an operation that consisted of removing a large piece of her skull on the left side. They put this piece in the freezer and will return it to here when the trauma in her brain is gone. Her neurosurgeon explained that this is a relatively new procedure which he and others in his field, especially in Germany, have pioneered. It is intended to relieve the pressure caused by the dead tissue on her left side. It prevents the damaged left side from inflicting damage on the right side of her brain. On Friday, even though the operation on Thursday was considered successful, there was a sudden increase in the intracranial pressure on the brain stem, which is "control center" for the brain. To relieve this pressure, the doctors had to go back in through the opening they had created on Thursday, and remove some of the damaged brain tissue in the left temporal lobe. They were also using medication to keep the pressure down. And they installed a pressure monitor in her brain. The pressure was maintained through Saturday, Sunday, and Monday. On Monday, they were able to remove the blood pressure monitor. They performed a test to see how bad the pressure could get, and it was within acceptable levels. On Tuesday they took her off the medication that was helping to maintain the blood pressure.

In cases of this kind, especially with the two surgeries, there is a significant danger of infection. No infection has occurred. There is also a danger of blood clots forming in other parts of her body, the lungs, etc. Again, none have occurred.

Beginning with the first surgery, Maureen has been kept sedated medicinally. On Sunday, they tried taking her off cold turkey and she reacted rather violently. This is a good sign. However, they put her back on sedation. On Monday, they again tried taking her off sedation, but this time gradually. On Tuesday, she was off sedation completely.

Along with removal of sedation, Maureen has shown good movement of her extremities. This has increased each day since Sunday. She is moving a lot on her left side, but there is also movement on her right side. Some of her right side movement is considered more than just reflex. If you put your hand in her left hand, she can squeeze quite strongly. She was opening her eyes on Tuesday.

Yesterday, Maureen showed the capability of responding to command. A doctor asked her to raise her left arm and she did. He told her to show two fingers. She showed three. He said, "I said two, not three," and she dropped one finger. Today, a nurse told her to lift her left leg to adjust her stocking. She did.

Another positive came up during her first neurological

examination last Wednesday. Maureen is apparently two-sided in regard to the part of the brain that initiates communication—thinking what you want to say before you say it. This occurs in only six percent of us.

And Maureen has a whole lot of family in the San Francisco area, most right here in the city. And she has many, many friends in the Bay Area, Los Angeles, Seattle, Washington, DC, New York, etc. Her e-mail list proves what a wealth of friends she has. And it goes further that that. My sister Mary Ann La Mere called our cousin Mary MacSweeney in Ireland. Mary Mac, as we call her, is the pipeline to our huge family in Ireland—more than 250 people. She is on my mother's side of the family. She called Donal Lehane, who is on my father's side, on his cell phone while he was in Lourdes in France. He is lighting candles for Maureen right there in the grotto.

Maureen has a long way to go. The medical staff cannot predict how far she can come back. But she is already showing signs of improvement. They are baby steps, but they are in the right direction. My wife Judy and I, Maureen's mother Pat Holmes, her brothers Kevin and Mike, her sister-in-law Joan, and all of the rest of the family are immensely thankful for your concern, your best wishes, your prayers, and your love for Maureen. We are all of us, friends and family together, of one mind in willing her speedy recovery. I will use this e-mail list to keep all of you informed of her progress.

—Jack Twomey

(Chapter 4)

June 14 or 15, my cousin Terry was
sitting by my bed reading from a
book of prayers. "What happened?" I
thought. "Is someone hurt? Hey . . . is
it me? In that case, I think it's minor."

Terri was crying. My mom,
Pat, was also reading something
inspirational and crying.

"Wait a minute . . . Is it worse?" I
wondered. "This must be a nightmare
. . . OH NO!"

Willie Twomey (Terri's brother)
was there too. He took my hand and
held it. I was so, so grateful to be
touching someone, and I thought, "If
you hold my hand, I will be okay."

Bridget gave the family a CD for me to have, Elliott Smith. In the note that accompanied it she wrote, "Maureen and I went to see Elliott Smith last Monday (June 5) at the Fillmore. Hopefully this will provide some good memories. Please Take Care, Bridget"

I think Elliott Smith should have come to see me on June 14 or later in 2000, to play songs for me. Shoot.

When Stephanie Barlow, my friend from Los Angeles (I met her at UCLA), got word from Heather Smith about what happened to me, she flew up and came to see me. She brought a photo album with pictures of me and other people in it to show me.

I had bandages that were constricting my body, and I didn't know what they were for. I wanted to take them off.

"Maureen, you have to keep them on," Stephanie told me. "I know they are uncomfortable, but they are preventing swelling."

I thought, "Ah, okay, I'll leave them on."

Sometimes it felt like a dream, and other times I STILL wasn't sure what was happening. I kept thinking, "Soon I'll wake up and I'll say, 'MAN, thank God I woke up!'"

I slept a LOT—so much so that I hadn't realized yet that I couldn't talk or walk. I thought I was just too tired. "I'll rest," I thought, "and then I'll say, 'Hey! I'm fine now! Where are my clothes? I want to get out of here.'"

I had no mirror, but the left side of my head felt like it was bald. "That's weird . . . oh! It must be a dream," I thought." It felt like there were flowers growing in my hair. Man, what a weird dream.

A little while later, some people came by, and I touched my head again. Wait . . . was I not dreaming? Half of my head WAS bald! But nobody was saying anything about it, so maybe no one had noticed there was something weird about my head except me. Hmmmmmm.

MaryAnn LaMere, my aunt, told me later that a lot of people knew about my head before they came to see me. "Remember!" other friends told them. "Don't mention Maureen's head!"

D'oh!

(I'm not sure when I also realized that some of my skull was missing; maybe June 24 or later? But thankfully I had bandages on my head at first. Sometime later the doctor removed the bandages. So if you saw me after I had the bandages off . . . sorry.)

Meanwhile, my neighbor William was still taking care of Salinger. (By the way, one of my favorite authors is J.D. Salinger; that's why I named her that.)

But now Salinger was scared: "Where is Maureen!?" she kept asking. (Well, she can't talk in English, but you could tell that's what she was thinking.)

William has a dog, which also scared Salinger, so finally he took her to Robert's place. Robert had two cats. William told me that Salinger was also scared of this new place at first, but they were taking good care of her.

Judy called the Avon Walk for Breast Cancer, saying what had happened to me and explaining why I could not go.

The woman said something like,

"Sorry, but she still pledged $2,500."

What?! (Did she think I was lying?!
"Oh I'm not sick at all, but I would
rather go on vacation instead." !!??!!)

Someone else quickly got on the
phone and told Judy she was so sorry
to hear what had happened to me, and
there was no need to give them the
money I'd pledged.

Gee, do you think?

Several e-mails from that time:

Date: June 16, 2000
From: Steve Beaumont (sbeaumont@...)
To: Mr. Twomey
Subject: Maureen

Mr. Twomey,

Your heartbreaking e-mail was sent to me by a friend
yesterday.

My name is Steve Beaumont. I was the creative director
at Ketchum Advertising in L.A. and Maureen's boss for two
years. My heart and prayers cry out to Maureen, you, and
her entire family.

Maureen's a beautiful, skilled, unique and interesting
person who helped herself to a promising creative career

through her own self-determination. Whatever luck she had, she created.

That this tragedy struck her so early in life, we are all deeply affected by the helplessness we feel for a friend. Secondly, as a father of a young adult woman, I can't imagine the grief you must have to endure during this time. I sense your courageousness reading your e-mails and know that Maureen is supported by a large and loving group of friends and family.

I first met Maureen working in our agency in the traffic department. At the time, she was interested in moving over to our creative department as a writer. Of course, people want to move over to the creative department all the time but Maureen had backed up her desire to write by actually writing radio commercials, magazine ads, TV spots. All fake, but they showcased her desire to be a copywriter. There was also another side to her that I felt would contribute to her success—a sarcastic, biting wit that manifested itself into impersonations of people, funny punch lines that were also poignant, and the occasional practical joke—like the outline of a dead body in masking tape on the floor outside her office to ward off any intruders. She used her skills to probe beneath the surface of a marketing problem, see through its veneer and communicate through her words in an honest, sometimes humorous, and direct way. We parted ways five years ago when I moved to another agency and she went to Chiat Day. I've followed the improving development of her work throughout the years and when I see her at industry functions, I always enjoy a sweet (sometimes sarcastic) hug and greeting based on mutual respect and admiration that we've earned from each other.

I'll also enjoy hearing of her progress because I know that underneath the surface, there's a free-spirited, strong-willed, determined woman fighting to get out and be heard. God bless Maureen and her family as you place her situation in His hands. May God comfort all and bring forward not only the best skills of the doctors, technicians, and support staff but all the love support and prayers of her friends and family as well.

Respectfully,
Steve Beaumont

....

From: Janet Kaspen (Perez)
Sent: June 14, 2000
To: KTwomey, Jack Twomey
Subject: From a friend

Dear Mr. Twomey:

My name is Janet Kasper and I've been friends with Maureen since we were both assistants at Rubin Postaer. Our friend Pete Gutzwiller has been forwarding your e-mails to me to keep me updated on Maureen.

Thank you so much for writing the letter updating us on her condition.

The e-mails you send are forwarded even farther to so many people pulling for Maureen. She is such an incredible person. Maureen has touched so many people with her keen wit and beautiful smile and wonderful friendship. It's our turn to touch her life with our prayers and good thoughts. We are all praying for her recovery and when she's ready, she'll be flooded with visitors to keep her company as she builds her journey through this time.

Please let her know that we all love her and are praying for her.

—Janet

....

From: Melanie K.
Sent: June 14, 2000
To: Kevin Twomey
Subject: Maureen

Dear Kevin,

I received the letter that your father sent to us about Maureen. My name is Melanie and I work at Goldberg Moser O'Neil. While I don't know Maureen very well, I know of her. I know that she is genuinely well liked and very talented.

I'm sure it is very hard for any of us to truly understand what your family must be going through. Your father's letter shed a little light on how difficult it must be for all of you, particularly Maureen. And about hope. And how we have to take it one day at a time.

I'm sending this letter to you to let you know that there are others here at GMO who like me, may not know a great deal about Maureen, but we have all been touched by what she is going through. She remains in our thoughts and in our hearts. I will continue to pray for her and to think positively as she continues to recover.

My heart goes out to you and your family.

—Melanie K.

From: Dean Poulakidas (UCLA)

Maureen is in my prayers, as are all of you—her family. Thank you for keeping us informed on her status.

—Dean Poulakidas

From: Monique Veillette

Thank you for the update. I will keep her in my prayers. It's great to hear she is doing better.

    Thank you so much for the letter. Please remember that I am only a few blocks from the hospital and at any time I am available to help in any way.

Thinking of all of you,
Monique

From: Amy C.
Sent: Thursday, June 15, 2000
To: Kevin Twomey

Hi Kevin,

My name is Amy C. and I am a co-worker of Maureen's. First let me say how sorry I am for everything she and your family has had to endure in the last week. It's wonderful to know she has such a large, supportive, and loving family. Thank you so much for forwarding your father's update.

As you know the entire agency is sending their prayers and best wishes.

I imagine you are trying to piece together all of the information prior to the stroke. And though I don't know how helpful I can be, I thought I should make myself available to you and your family.

I was the person who first found Maureen on Tuesday. I called her doctor and then 911 and tried to comfort her while we waited for the paramedics. I also gave them as much information as I could as to what happened from the time I discovered her (just moments after she collapsed). I was unable to go to the hospital with her, but thankfully, Noreen, as you know, accompanied her to the hospital.

I don't know if it would be helpful, but if you'd like to contact me for any reason, please feel free to do so: home: _____ work: _____.

Please know that I haven't stopped thinking about or sending Maureen my positive thoughts since Tuesday. She is such a strong and wonderful woman. I am praying for her daily progress.

With my very best wishes,
Amy

....

June 16, 2000
Dear Friends of Maureen,

Maureen has been making fantastic progress the last two days. Last Sunday she was on six "drips." Now she is down to one, the feeding tube into her nose. She is completely off of the oxygen machine, breathing on her own. She is coughing and needs some suction (just like in the dentist's chair) occasionally to recover from the complications of being on oxygen.

She makes the sort of eye-to-eye contact that makes you feel that she really knows who you are. When you come in to see her, she looks at you strongly, and when you put your hand in her left hand, she squeezes strongly.

I picked up her portable CD player at her apartment and brought it into ICU. When I put the headphones on her, she reached up with her left hand and adjusted the headphone so that she could hear better. After listening to a few cuts, she tired a little; so she reached up and took the headphones off.

The nurses made up a sign with "Yes" on one side and "No" on the other. They show it to her, ask a question, and she points to the answer she wants. So she can see, she can read, she can hear and she can choose her response.

Today Maureen is being moved from Medical-Surgical ICU to Transitional ICU. She is no longer on the "critical" list. They are trying to get her a room with a window, so that she can gaze upon the mansions of Pacific Heights and perhaps the greenery of Lafayette Park. When I see her later today, I will find out what sort of rules they have in TICU for visiting, etc.

—Jack Twomey

(Well, I guess I figured out what "Yes"
and "No" meant; but most other words
I didn't. Not for a while.)

(Chapter 5)

Friday, June 16, 2000

Now I could see outside. Well, I was
INside, but still.

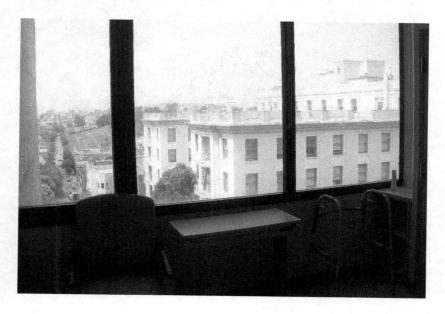

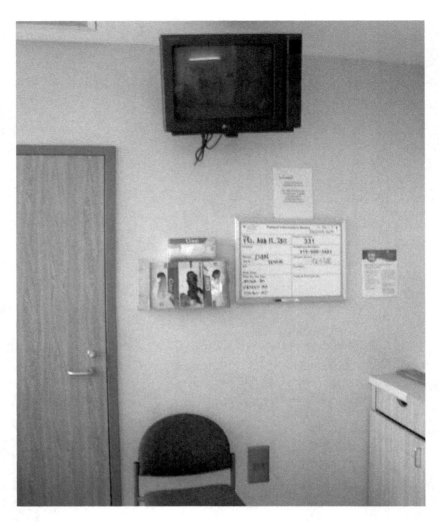

(I couldn't see on my right, but I
didn't realize that because the window
was on my left. On the right side of
my bed, there was only a curtain.)

It was cloudy but it was daytime
. . . ahhhhhhh. I nodded off. When I
woke up, it was still daytime. I nodded

off again . . . woke up and it was still daytime . . .

Now I was kind of irritated. It was still cloudy, so I couldn't tell what time it was. "Is it 10:00 a.m.? 2:30 p.m.? 7:45 p.m.? !#%*@!"

I love summertime, but I was inside and doing NOTHING except for lying in bed. No one was in my room; but even if someone was there, I couldn't say "Hey, what time is it?" because I couldn't TALK! Aaaaaaaaaaaaah!

Finally, the sun came out. But now it was so bright that I could hardly see. Some nurse came in, and she noticed I was squinting. She said something like, "Do you want me to close the blinds?"

I nodded yes. Man . . . she was psychic!

Another time the TV was on in my room and I wanted it off. (In junior-high, we had a TV – you could make it off, low, medium, high, and off again.) So I tried to turn it off, but it only got louder and louder and LOUDER! "How do I turn it off?!" I wondered.

I was alone—the nurse was not
in my room—and I couldn't talk, so I
was helpless. Aaaaaaaaah!

Maybe it was so loud that
everyone could hear it in the hall, I
don't know, but finally the nurse came
to check on me. I tried to tell her
that I wanted to turn the TV off. She
understood and turned it off.

"THANK YOU!" I thought.
"*Aaaahhhhh*, thank you . . .
thank you . . . zzzzzzzzzzz"

My cousin, Kathy Looney, and my
Aunt Eileen came to visit me.

Later, Kathy told me that she
knew I couldn't talk, but she sensed
that I was fully aware. So she knew I
had not turned to mush.

. . . Thanks Kathy?

(Chapter 6)

Monday, June 19, 2000

I moved to a new room.

I still thought I was just too tired to read words. "When I'm better," I thought, "I'll be able to read them again."

So they gave me this chart so I could tell them what I was saying:

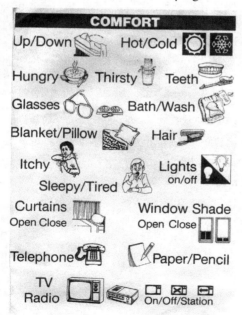

("Haaa! Yeah right," I thought later—

'I want to call someone'? 'Can you give me some paper and a pencil; I will tell you what I mean' . . . !?)

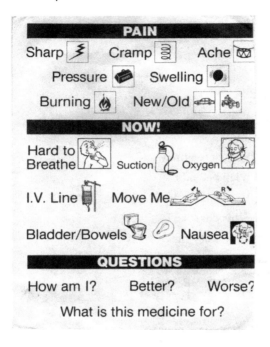

"The Critical Communicator"
Here's the website:
http://www.alimed.com/the-critical-communicator.html

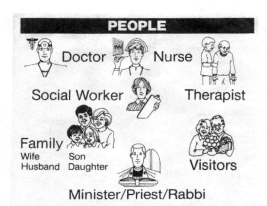

PEOPLE

Doctor Nurse

Social Worker Therapist

Family
Wife Son
Husband Daughter
Visitors

Minister/Priest/Rabbi

PERSONALIZED NEEDS/WORDS

YES   NO

A B C D E F G H
I J K L M N O P Q
R S T U V W X Y Z
1 2 3 4 5 6 7 8 9 0

JANUARY	MONDAY	
FEBRUARY		
MARCH	TUESDAY	
APRIL		
MAY	WEDNESDAY	
JUNE		
JULY	THURSDAY	
AUGUST		
SEPTEMBER	FRIDAY	
OCTOBER	SATURDAY	Day ☀ Night 🌙
NOVEMBER		
DECEMBER	SUNDAY	Morning/Afternoon/Evening

interactive
THERAPEUTICS, INC.™ P.O. BOX 1805, STOW, OHIO 44224 1-800-253-5111 FAX: 330-923-3030

Critical Communicator
PRODUCT #170
© 1993 Interactive Therapeutics, Inc. All Rights Reserved.

Dad wrote on June 14,

"She has lost vision on the right side in both eyes . . ."

When I was on the west side of the hospital, in my first room, my right side faced the curtain, and the window was on my left. So it didn't occur to me that I couldn't see on my right side.

My new room, on the east side of the hospital, was bigger. From my bed I could see nurses, doctors, etc. outside on my left. I could see the TV set was square in the middle. But if I was looking at the TV set, I couldn't see anything on the right . . .

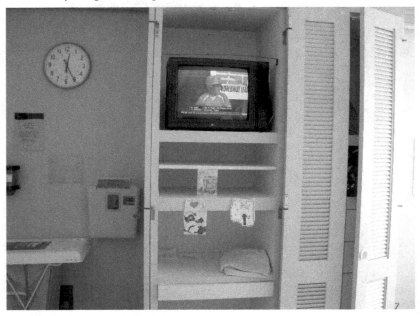

. . . So I turned some more to
the right, then I could finally see the
window:

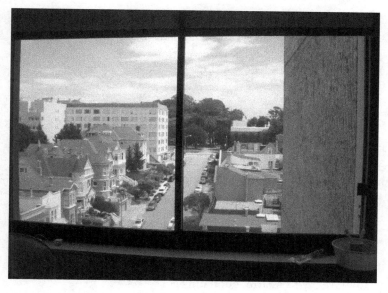

"That's strange!" I thought. "I can
see with both eyes, so why can't I see
the window?" (This is when I knew that
there was a problem with my eyes!)

I got my first real food on Tuesday,
June 20. I think they gave me gelatin
first. I tried to eat it, but,

a) I use to be right-handed, and
this was my first time trying to use a
fork with my left hand; and

b) gelatin is hard to do with your weak hand. I think I only managed to get one or two bites in my mouth . . . d'oh!

So they gave me pudding instead. Mmmmmm . . . so much better.

It was 6:00 p.m. or so, and the nurses were talking outside my room. My right arm was asleep, and stuck behind me, and I couldn't get it back in front. I should have just used my left arm to help, and it would have been all better. But I didn't think about that. I tried to move my right arm, but it only got more stuck.

One nurse came in and said, "Oh my gosh. Why are you twisted around like that? How did you get like that?"

("Obviously, I can't tell you," I thought. "Just help me.")

Someone else came in and the two of them helped me get untangled.

From: Lisa Motel
Sent: Wednesday, June 2000
To: Kevin Twomey, Jack Twomey
Subject: Ever MORE Love than you know

Dear Mr. Twomey,

I know your daughter from her first job at Ketchum Advertising when she began as a traffic manager, before she unleashed her talent as a writer. It has been a number of years since I have seen her but I have kept tabs on her career at Chiat Day and at Goldberg Moser O'Neil.

I have been forwarded your memo regarding Maureen. Unbelievable this test for her and for the closest ones who love her.

The family of loving human beings is far and wide. There are hundreds of us sending prayers for the speediest recovery possible and a full healing of body and spirit.

I ask G-d that he show us the power of our prayer. That Maureen will triumph back to live a life with mobility and freedom. May G-d grant many miracles for her and your family.

Please know that I have forwarded via e-mail, Maureen's medical situation to my Jewish Spiritual Community. We will all pray for her and for you. Together with the hundreds of others—from all theology and background, with the love that makes us all the same family. Heaven is hearing from US.

You are not alone.

—Lisa Motel

Really late Tuesday or really early Wednesday morning, June 20/21, 2000:

Soon there was another accident. I was dreaming about sheets. (Other people dream about much better things. I dream about sheets . . . ?)

In the dream, I was going to pick out the sheets I wanted. Then I thought, "I should get up; so many other people are sicker then me, so I will give the bed to someone else who needs it more." So I was going to get up and leave, but I couldn't get up. I tried it again . . . why can't I get up?! Well, I guess I finally got out of bed . . . and immediately fell down on the floor.

A nurse was outside the room and heard the noise. She came in and saw what was going on, and she and somebody else helped me get in the bed again.

After that, they put a tube inside my nose that would set off an alarm if it happened again. It was like I was a convict.

When morning came, a nurse gave my breakfast and I tried to eat it, but the tube got in the way. AAAAAAAAH!

"Can someone take it out," I thought?

The doctor came to my room. "I know it's uncomfortable," she said, "but you could fall of the bed again or something worse. Give it some time, and we will see how you're doing then . . ." ☹

(Chapter 7)

June 22, 2000

In the morning, Dad and two other
people came to fill out some forms.

DURABLE FOR POWER OF ATTORNEY
FOR PROPERTY AND HEALTH CARE
APPOINTMENT OF ATTORNEY IN FACT

I, Maureen Ellen Twomey, a resident of San Francisco, California, appoint my father, John A. Twomey, as my attorney in fact for the purposes of managing my property and financial affairs from the date of execution of this document, and my health care decisions in the event that I become incapacitated and cannot make health care decision on my own. This Durable Power of Attorney is executed by me on this day of 6/22/2000, at San Francisco, California.

✗ ☐

_____

Maureen Ellen Twomey

(Of course, I didn't write this. My Dad wrote it; I just checked the box above my name.) Then the two other people signed and dated it.

In the afternoon, I finally realized, that I was not just really tired; that I could no longer walk, talk, read, or write . . . but because I'd had a huge, huge, HUGE stroke

. . . I couldn't walk at all
BECAUSE I'D HAD A STROKE
. . . I couldn't speak at all
BECAUSE I'D HAD A STROKE
. . . I couldn't read and write at all
BECAUSE I'D HAD A STROKE . . .

AAAAA
AAAAA
AAAAA
AAAHH
HHHHH
HHHHH
!!!!!!!!!!

Why? Why?
Why???????!!!!!!!

AAAAA
AAAAH
HHHHH
HHHHH!

(CHAPTER 8)

June 23, 2000
Dear Friends of Maureen,

I meant to send another note quicker than this, but . . . Last Friday, June 16, Maureen was moved from Medical Surgical ICU to Transitional ICU. She stayed there until Monday. Then she was moved into a regular part of the hospital, 5 North. Her room is ___. It is quite large and has a nice view of Lafayette Park, plus a TV, stereo, a VCR if she wants one, etc. Clearly, she is a whole lot better. Wednesday evening, she had her first meal . . .

(Well, Tuesday, June 20, I had gelatin/
pudding. Wednesday the 21st, I had my
first real meal, I guess.)

. . . The doctors have been conducting what they call "swallow studies" each day after leaving TICU. By Wednesday, they thought that she could have pureed foods and thick liquids. Her dinner included chocolate pudding, which she enjoyed immensely, feeding herself quite well with her left hand. There was also a vanilla flavored shake-sort-of-thing that she drank through a straw. However, the main course was pureed pork chop with mushrooms. One spoonful was enough; the look on her face was a clear "Ugh!" They continue with the NG tube to make sure that she gets the nutrient she needs. And they will continue with their "swallow studies" until they are sure that she can safely handle thin liquids like water and champagne. Just kidding! She is also showing a small smile at times and appears to understand a lot of what is said to her.

The medical staff is keeping an attendant in her room because Maureen crawled out of bed Tuesday night. They found her on the floor tangled in her support lines. Apparently, she suffered no further harm. She could have, since the left side of her brain is unprotected. Most people think that her attempt shows a spirit that will do her well in recuperation.

Maureen has been receiving physical therapy and speech therapy. They are just at the initial stages, doing what seem like simple things, but of course are not so simple to her. She has been sitting in a chair, standing up with support, things like that.

The visiting rules are much more flexible than in ICU. Maureen's room is large and can accommodate more than just a couple of people. There is a large and well-furnished waiting room close by. The medical staff said that they would like visitors to be quiet when in the hallways since noise can affect other patients. Otherwise, use your judgment. If there are other friends or family visiting Maureen, work out something sensible. The hospital is California Pacific Medical Center at Buchanan and Clay Streets in San

Francisco. Her room number again is ___. As you get off the elevator, go left.

Thanks for all of the wonderful expressions of concern for Maureen. It is awful hard to discourage her friends from sending flowers, but, if I could get you all together in one huge room, I would be able to pick out one small group and say "Okay, you guys can send the flowers. That'll take care of the flowers. Everybody else can do something else, send a card, or a note, or whatever else you think of." Maureen's friends at Goldberg, Moser, O'Neill asked if Maureen would appreciate a blood drive in her honor. Even though she has not needed a lot of blood transfusions, I was able to assure them that Maureen would indeed appreciate it. She has been donating blood herself on a regular basis.

—Jack and Judy Twomey

Some friends came to see me. One woman said,

"D O   Y O U
W A N T   U S
T O   T A L K
S L O W E R,
S O   Y O U
C A N   H E A R
E V E R Y -
T H I N G
W E   S A Y ?"

"Aaaaaaaah!" I thought.

Thankfully someone else said, "She can totally understand everything you say, so you don't have to talk slower—SHE just can't talk."

"Thank you," I thought. "Everyone else can talk. You be quiet."

(Sorry lady . . . I'm having a lousy day.)

Some time later, a woman said that I was so strong—she said something like, "I would never be so strong."

"But," I thought, "I didn't want to be in this thing, not ever! I'm the same as you, but it happened to me. Do you really think I'm braver then you?"

❀ ❀ ❀

June 24, 2000

Mom and my improv people were visiting (Laura Derry, Jennifer, and some more). One of the improv people was telling a story, but my mom kept interrupting.

So I said my first words, and they were . . . "BUTT OUT!"

(Or "SHUT UP!" . . . I can't actually remember which two words I said.)

My mom said, "YEEEEAAAAHHH!! You can

talk! I don't care what you call
me! But you can TALK NOW!
YEEEEEAAAAHHH!!!"

I was still mad at my mom ... I
didn't realize that I could finally talk,
I just wanted her to shut up. I thought
she was laughing at me.

When the improv people were
gone, I said my second words: "MOM
... GO!"

(Sorry, Mom.)

Much later, MaryAnn told me
about when she was a nurse and some
male nurse she worked with was
taking care of a patient who couldn't
talk at all. I don't think the nurse was
even bugging the patient; he was just
seeing if he needed anything: "Can
I get anything for you? Do you need
something?"

So the first words that the patient
said were: "When are you going on
vacation?"

Haaa!

❀   ❀   ❀

I think the third thing I said was
"apple," the next day, in reference to
some apple sauce. My friend Suzanne
was there.

I had somewhat lost my short-term memory, so I often couldn't remember something five or ten seconds after it happened.

If I was in the room alone and I wanted to ask for something to drink . . . when someone came in, I would know I needed to say something, so I'd just say "orange juice," even if I really didn't want that, just because I couldn't name anything else.

There were times when they brought me something and insisted that I had asked for it when I was sure I had actually asked for something else. "I clearly know what I wanted," I thought . . . but hmmmm, maybe not. Some definitions of the things I had:

ACQUIRED DYSGRAPHIA: Dysgraphia acquired as a result of brain damage or injury.

APHASIA: An acquired language disorder caused by brain damage with complete or partial impairment of language, comprehension, formulation, or use. ▶

APRAXIA: A speech disorder in which the person cannot control the speech muscles and movements in order to intentionally produce specific phonemes or connected speech.

COGNITIVE DEFICITS: Cognition is the act or process of knowing including awareness and judgment. The characteristics that serve as a barrier to cognitive performance are called cognitive deficits. For example, difficulty in processing phonological information is a cognitive deficit that has a negative impact of the development of reading skill.

Great.

The Brain ...

Left brain	vs.	Right brain
Verbal		Non-verbal
Logic		Emotion
Reasoning		Intuition
Speech		Imagination
Writing		Daydreaming
Objectivity		Big Picture
Linear		Spatial

Math	Subjectivity
Science	Melody
Analytic	Creative

(etc.)

Before I had a stroke, some teachers tested me, and my brain was mostly equally spread: 53% left and 47% right.

I didn't undergo the same tests after my stroke, but I think my brain was more like this:

Left: 4%
Right: 96%
   (Non-verbal: 40%)
   (Emotion: 27%)
   (Daydreaming: 27%)
   (Other: 6%)

That's what it felt like, anyway.

(Chapter 9)

I "worked" with Terry Jew, a physical therapist (PT), and Geary Shew, an occupational therapist (OP), every day.

I was so tired. "Come on, Maureen," Terry said. "You have to get better, you have to exercise."

So we ran a half-marathon.

Just kidding . . .we did basic stuff like sitting in a chair, moving from the chair to a wheelchair, then moving back out of the wheelchair and into the chair again.

I still had my apartment, but I didn't know when I would go home. My apartment building had no elevator.

I lived on the third floor; now that I couldn't walk, that was a problem.

So my dad and some friends moved my stuff out of my apartment and into storage.

The manager of the building said she was "so sorry" to hear about what happened to me. "Me too," I thought. :-l

I got many cards wishing me good thoughts and prayers. I couldn't read at all, but I couldn't talk much at all on the phone, either, so friends wrote me notes and my family and friends read them to me when they came to visit.

GMO (now GMO/Hill Holliday) gave me a HUGE picture of me (not a picture of me in the hospital; it was me at work in May 2000). Someone made a poster for me, too, and everyone signed it (so again, someone else read it to me later).

Jenn Muranaka-Chaney and a lot of other people at TBWA\Chiat\Day made a video for me:

In case you haven't figured it out, the "MIA copywriter" is me. It ended with:

"CREATED WITH LOVE
FROM YOUR FRIENDS AT
CHAIT/DAY
AND SMITH/NELSON"

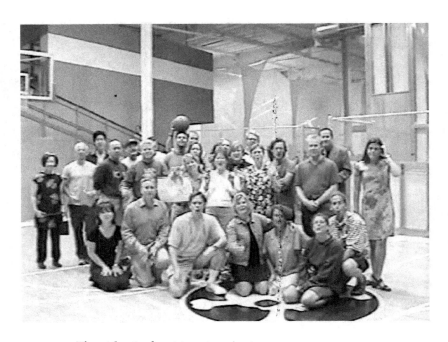

The video is about twenty minutes
or so long. It starts with a lot of people
saying "WHOOOHOOOOO!!"
and then goes on to show a lot of
people wishing me good thoughts.
One of them was from Lee Clow, "Hi
Maureen, this is Lee. I know you're not
working anymore here, but damn it,
I'm sort of your boss – get better ..." ☺

Another one from Hank: "Maureen,
kick the therapist. You'll feel better."

(Whoever is reading this and is
a therapist, rest assured he was just
kidding . . . I think so, anyway.)

❀ ❀ ❀

I still had the tube in my nose, so
eating food was uncomfortable—the
tube always got in the way.

"If you eat more, Maureen, maybe
I can take your tube out," a doctor said.

"But it's so uncomfortable that I
can't eat!" I thought. "Aaaaaah! It's a
vicious cycle!!"

❀ ❀ ❀

On the Fourth of July, friends and
family came to see me. When people
began to leave, I got depressed. "Take
me with you!" I thought.

By about 7:00 p.m., everyone
was gone. I was thinking about my
apartment and wishing I could be
there to watch the fireworks that night.

I took a nap, and at 9:30 p.m. I
woke up to the sound of fireworks
galore going off. I think if you're higher
up at the hospital in the west or north
side, you can see the fireworks from
the windows. But I was looking out the
east side of the building. Darn it!

❀ ❀ ❀

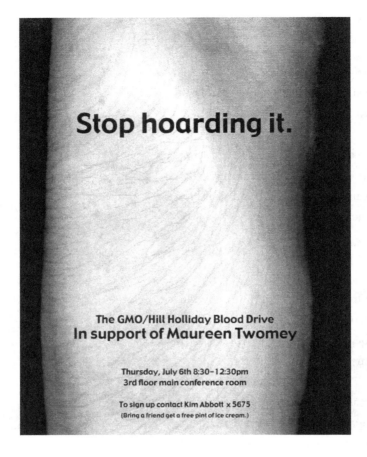

Stop hoarding it.

The GMO/Hill Holliday Blood Drive
In support of Maureen Twomey

Thursday, July 6th 8:30–12:30pm
3rd floor main conference room

To sign up contact Kim Abbott x 5675
(Bring a friend get a free pint of ice cream.)

Thanks! And if you ever need
some blood, call me.

July 9, 2000

They finally took the tube out of my
nose today . . . YEAH!!! I was so
grateful.

(Later I realized I should have kept my nose tube and framed it. Oh well.)

After they took out the tube, they gave me lunch. The doctor said, "Remember, you have to eat more food at every meal now." The lunch was spaghetti with a whole lot of onions . . . I don't like onions, but I was so happy to finally be able to eat that I didn't care.

Thankfully, soon after that my friends Lauren Harwell (Godfrey), Bridget, Maya Seely, Sarah Glicken, and Monique Veillette brought me real food (pizza!) from outside. Thaaaaaaaaaaaank you!

I thought the hospital food people should call the pizza place and say, "Can you cater every day now? Because Maureen Twomey would like that."

9 July 2000

Dear Friends of Maureen,

My son Kevin is on vacation. I have been relying on him to forward these letters to Maureen's friends. I got a copy of her list and finally have the ball rolling. I will not bore you will all the complication that delayed this.

Maureen is definitely getting better and better. In the last two weeks, she has fought off two staph infections. Today she is running a slight temperature that is related to the second infection, so she is still getting antibiotics intravenously. The medical staff said that the staph infection has been identified as one of those that is treatable by antibiotics. And that is all of the news that is not good (there is no really bad news).

For the good news, Maureen is starting to speak again. I received two versions of her first words. The first version, although apparently not accurate, is a classic. This was on Saturday, June 24. According to this version, some friends of Maureen from her Improv group were visiting along with her Mom. The group were doing a skit that Maureen had practiced with them. During the recreation, Maureen's Mom was reported to horn in a little bit, and Maureen is supposed to have said, "Mom, butt out!" When I later heard a second version, the Improv group had already left, but two of the medical staff heard Maureen say "Mom, go" and then "but . . ."

Next on Thursday, June 29, Suzanne B. heard Maureen say "apple," asking for applesauce. Now, Maureen is regularly saying "yes" and "no" and "Hi!" and a few other words, beginning the long slow course back to regular conversation.

Maureen was taken off of the NG feeding tube today. She is really happy about that. She had a real chocolate milk shake from Swensen's as part of her lunch today. The positive aspect of the NG tube was that it guaranteed that she had all of the nutrients that she needed. Now she is going to have to eat a balanced diet so that she can stay healthy.

There are even a few small positive signs regarding her right-hand side. We have noticed that the right side of her face does not show the drop that is apparent with some people who have suffered stroke. And the physical therapist has said that there are positive indications.

All of this progress means that Maureen will be leaving the hospital soon. Most probably she will then go to a rehabilitation facility. However, we have learned that the doctors are not into long term or even medium term planning. They still have a day by day approach. They want her to be in a stable medical condition before taking the next step.

Thank you all for your concern, the beautiful flowers, the cute gifts, the many visits to Maureen, and for the voicemail messages set up by Alison Van Dyke (650-___-____).

Jack & Judy Twomey

My friend Alison Van Dyke had put
a message on a voicemail service
for me so you could call and leave
a message for me: "Welcome to
Maureen's voicemail, where you can
leave your positive thoughts, and get
well messages. The system may cut
you off at three minutes, so feel free to
call back, and call back as much as you
want, because Maureen would love to
hear from you. Thanks for calling!"
    It was SOOOO nice of her to
think of this idea!
    One message from my friend

Morgan Rumpf: "Hey Maureen, this is Morgan . . . HONEY! Hi, don't think you're not getting out of your Christmas card this year, you know because of this health stuff . . . (kidding). I look forward to your Christmas card every year, and I want it to be especially creative this year! So anyway, I just thought I call and say hi . . ."

That was just one of maaaaany other voicemails left for me by my friends.

(Sorry, I would give the number to YOU, so you could leave a message for me too, but now it's no longer in service. Darn.)

(Chapter 10)

The hospital people—nurses, doctors, physical therapists, etc.—were so nice and so great at their jobs.

One, however, was so unkind. One day I wanted to say something, and I was struggling for words, but she was impatient. She seemed like she could care less. I was seriously hurt, and she could see how sick I was. "I'm trying to explain," I thought, "but you keep interrupting!"

She said something like, "What do you want?" in an impatient tone. "If you can't get your words out," she told me, "I'm busy."

I was irritated with her now, and upset. So I tried to do it myself (I can't remember what it was) . . . and she started laughing at me!! AAAAAAAH!

I thought, "You're a nurse. Nurses are supposed to be patient. You go into the job not because the people in the hospital are going to say thank you. Maybe you can do the job a nurse can do, but if you are not in love with your job . . . you're not sensitive and caring. You're just anxious to finish your shift. You might have to stay overtime because there are sick people here who need help— that's part of your job. I would do this myself if I could, but I can't."

Actually, I can't remember if that nurse was ever in my room again, so maybe she was just having one bad day. If that's the case, I apologize to YOU, lady.

Some UCLA friends, Wendy Law, Luis Ramos, Anya, and other people came to see me. They made cards for me so I could communicate better, including these:

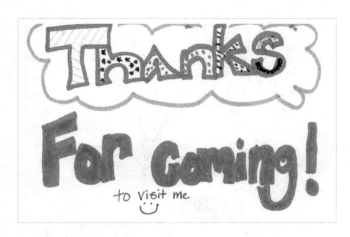

Thanks For coming!
to visit me ☺

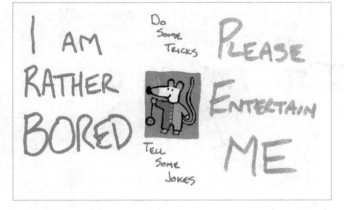

I AM RATHER BORED

Do Some Tricks

Tell Some Jokes

PLEASE Entertain ME

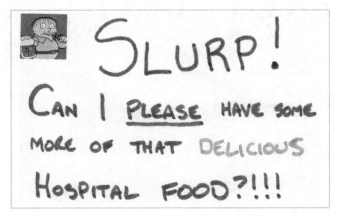

SLURP!

CAN I PLEASE HAVE SOME MORE OF THAT DELICIOUS HOSPITAL FOOD?!!!

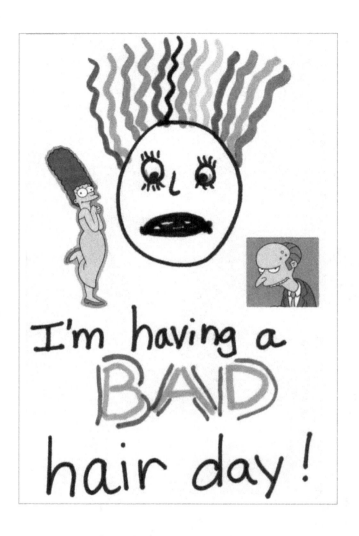

. . . HEY! I'm NOT having a bad
hair day!!

("Yes, Maureen, you ARE.")

❀　❀　❀

Sometime in July 2000, Dr. Kitt came to visit me, and he brought his young daughters. He said he was so happy that I was doing so much better; he hadn't thought I was going to make it, and he wanted to have his girls come and see how much better I was.

Dr. Rome, who was in charge of rehab at Davies Campus, came to see me and assessed my case. He said he thought I would make a good candidate for rehab. When he told me that, I thought, "I'm in! I will be 100 percent better in four weeks! WHOOHOOOOOO!"

(I thought . . .)

Every week they weighed me at 6:00 a.m. or so. I couldn't walk, so a guy transferred me to a cot, and then he lifted me up and THEN he weighed me. It was SOOOO excruciating! AAAAAH! I felt like only my middle sections were secured when he lifted me, because my head and legs were limp. I would attempt to lift my head so my head and my middle were level, but I couldn't.

The picture below shows what it looked like, except that in 2000, there was no armrest that I could use to sit up when they weighed me. (I can't find a picture that has no armrest, so just pretend there isn't one.

That's me:

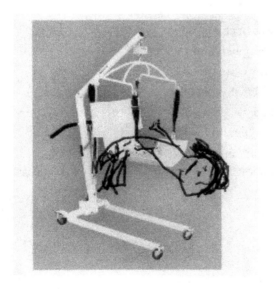

"Wow Maureen, you draw exceptionally well!" (Not.)

They never told me how much I weighed. If I had asked them I'm sure they would have told me, but the only thing I was thinking was, "GET ME DOWN!! AAAAAAH!"

Mostly I had no exercise; I was just eating and sleeping. I'm 5'6," and I had weighed 118 pounds before the stroke. I thought I must have gained tons of weight since it happened. But later, in rehab, they weighed me again (THANKFULLY there was an armchair, so I got to sit up), and I found out I was only 104 pounds. "Aaaaaah! I'm so thin!" (Not a good thin.) "Eat, Maureen! Eat!"

I got a new helmet. I still couldn't walk alone, but I had to wear it when anyone was helping me out of the bed and into the wheelchair, etc.

I was almost out of the hospital and about to go to rehab when I developed a huge allergic skin rash. Great.

19 July 2000
Dear Friends of Maureen,

There has been a lot of progress, if you measure in small steps. Maureen is still getting antibiotics. It is hard to determine whether there is still some real infection or whether the medical staff is just being prudent, maybe overly prudent. In any event, Maureen is doing better.

She is saying more and more. She has a command of a lot of the little words that surround the more meaningful words, but has trouble getting out those more meaningful words that express the idea. But she is trying. Sometimes you feel that the frustration would stifle the attempt, but she is trying. Tonight she was in really good spirits in spite of the fact that it does not always work as well as you would like.

Last Sunday I offered to get some food for Maureen from outside the hospital. I asked her if she would like some ravioli. And she heartily agreed. After I got it, she enjoyed it immensely. On Tuesday, my sister Mary Ann and her husband Chuck were visiting and asked her if she wanted some outside food. They made several suggestions and then Chuck gave her a pad of paper and a pen. She wrote out "RAV." This is the first time that she has communicated by writing since her stroke. A small beginning.

I have only a few memorable things on the walls of my office at work. One is a quote from a Frenchman who said, "The distance was nothing. Only the first step was difficult." It then goes on to explain that he was talking about the story that St. Denis, the patron saint of France, was reputed to have walked six miles carrying his severed head in his hands. Only the first step was difficult! For Maureen, it may not be quite as dramatic, but you do feel that the first steps rapidly grow to a certain, swift recuperation.

Maureen is still at California Pacific Medical Center hospital at Buchanan and Clay. Her doctors have decided to move her to the Acute Rehabilitation center at the California Pacific Davies center at Duboce and Castro. They are waiting for a bed to become vacant. This facility has a very good reputation.

She is buoyed by all of the kind notes and cards and remembrances that she is getting from all of her friends.

—Jack and Judy Twomey

(Chapter 11)

Finally . . . Rehab at Davies Campus:
July (21?) →

    (I use to be right-handed; this is
my left hand below.)

Reference

Subject: Medical History

Type of injury: STROKE

Date of injury: JUNE 6 2000

Dates of hospitalization: JUNE 6 2000

Name of hospital: CPMC

Location of hospital: DAVIES

Surgeries: CRANIOTOMY
LOBECTOMY (TEMPORAL LOBE)

Therapy received:	Therapists:
Physical	Denise
Speech	Kalina
occupational	Joanie

Physicians: Dr Ng , Dr. Patrick Tekeli
Dr Osterweil (Neuropsychology)

I just copied this; I mostly couldn't read yet, so Kalynn, the speech person, helped me. Here is the "real" one:

CALIFORNIA PACIFIC MEDICAL – DAVIES CAMPUS, 7/25/00

CONSULTATION PHYSICAL MEDICANE REFERRING: STEPHEN NG, M.D.

REHABILITATION TEAM CONFERENCE

DISCHARGE: END DATE IS AUGUST 18, 2000
(4 weeks)

SELF-CARE:

EATING: THE PATIENT IS MINIMAL ASSIST.
GROOMING: THE PATIENT IS MINIMAL ASSIST.
BATHING: THE PATIENT IS MODERATE ASSIST.
DRESSING BODY: THE PATIENT IS MINIMAL/
MODERATE ASSIST.

TRANSFERS:

BED, CHAIR, WHEELCHAIR, BED AND SHOWER TRANSFERS: THE PATIENT IS MODERATE ASSIST.

LOCOMOTION:

WALKING AND STAIR TAKING: THE PATIENT IS TOTALLY DEPENDENT.

COMMUNICATION:

COMPREHENS: THE PATIENT IS MODERATE ASSIST.
EXPRESSION: THE PATIENT IS MAXIMAL ASSISTANCE.

SOCIAL COGNITION:

SOCIAL INTERACTION: THE PATIENT IS MINIMAL ASSIST.

PROBLEM SOLVING: THE PATIENT IS MODERATE ASSIST.

MEMORY: THE PATIENT IS MODERATE ASSIST.

—STEPHEN NG, M.D.

I could finally look in the mirror. Part of the left side of my head was still gone. That was no longer a shock to me. The part that had been removed was stored in a freezer. When the swelling was completely healed, the doctors would put it back. In the meantime I wore my helmet all the time; I only took it off when I took a shower (duh) and when I was in bed (duh again).

(Much later I thought, "Hey, I should have gone to 7-11 with the helmet on my head, gotten two six-packs of beer, and seen if they needed to see my ID card. Oh well.")

In TV or soap operas, people in bed look perfect; maybe they have bandages on, but a week later, they're fine. Well, I also looked perfect . . . yeah right.

In the CPCH I had my own room. When I came to Davies Campus, I had two other people in the room with me. It was a big room, and you could draw the curtains, but you could still hear other conversations. Some people talked quieter (thank you); some other people talked louder, but that didn't really bother me either. The only thing I don't like is really loud snoring. Thankfully, the two other people in my room didn't snore.

I had a wheelchair, but I could only push with my left leg and left arm. "Great, I can't go fast in the wheelchair. Shoot."

I still had a rash all over my body . . . rrrrrrr. I looked like a snake whose skin was peeling. I think other people must have thought, "She has so much dandruff!" :-l

I couldn't see on the right side, so one day I bumped into somebody who was also in a wheelchair during lunch in the rec room. "Whoops! I apologize!" And I rolled on. The old man I'd run into was stunned.

Anyway, back to the important stuff. Every day I worked with three people: Denise Hong, a physical therapist (PT); Kalynn, a speech therapist; and Joanie Hooper, an occupational therapist (OP).

I thought if I worked hard
and participated in rehab, I'd be
100 percent better in four weeks.
Whoohooo!

Every day, Joanie came and
helped me get out of the wheelchair
and into the bath chair so I could
shower alone. (At CPMC, they had
mostly helped me do it.) When I was
done, Joanie helped me back into the
wheelchair.

I could finally wear my own
clothes. The first day, I put on a pretty
dress and formal pumps (after all, I
had to make a good impression!).

HAAA! Just kidding about the
dress. I wore comfortable clothes that
I could wear when I was doing PT
and OP.

Some OP exercises I did with
Joanie:

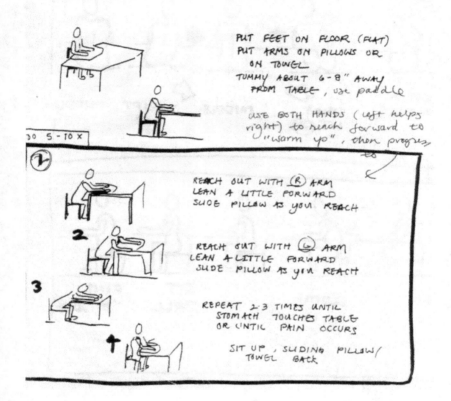

DO ALL EXERCISES TO POINT OF STRETCH (NOT PAIN)

PUT FEET ON FLOOR (FLAT)
PUT ARMS ON PILLOWS OR
   ON TOWEL
TUMMY ABOUT 6 - 8" AWAY
   FROM TABLE, use paddle

USE BOTH HANDS (left helps right) to reach forward to "warm up", then progress

DO 5 - 10 X

1. REACH OUT WITH (R) ARM
LEAN A LITTLE FORWARD
SLIDE PILLOW AS YOU REACH

2. REACH OUT WITH (L) ARM
LEAN A LITTLE FORWARD
SLIDE PILLOW AS YOU REACH

3. REPEAT 2-3 TIMES UNTIL
STOMACH TOUCHES TABLE
OR UNTIL PAIN OCCURS

SIT UP, SLIDING PILLOW/
   TOWEL BACK

Kalynn was my speech as well as my reading/writing person. The following items are the things we worked on together (I couldn't read these yet, but I think everyone else can, including you):

Word finding Strategies

1. Gesture
2. Description-function
3. Visualization
4. Give Maureen the first sound of the word.

Feelings

O.K-Okay
Great
Bad
Tired
Sad
Happy
Angry
Frustrated
Pain
Anxious

Body parts

Waist

Hips

Knee

Ankle

Leg

Toes

Foot

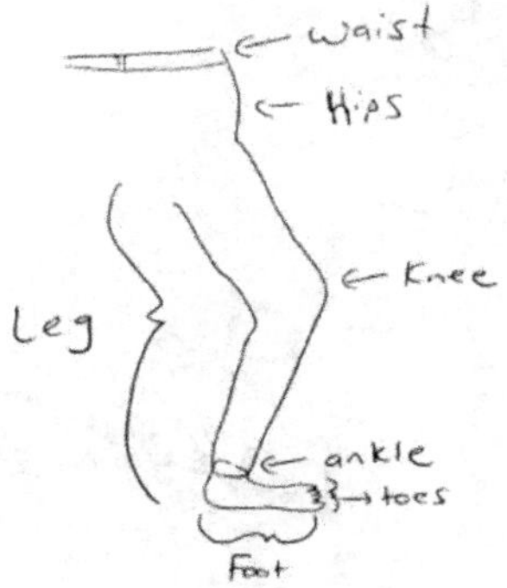

ELBOW

SHOULDER

THUMB

FINGERS

WRIST

ARM

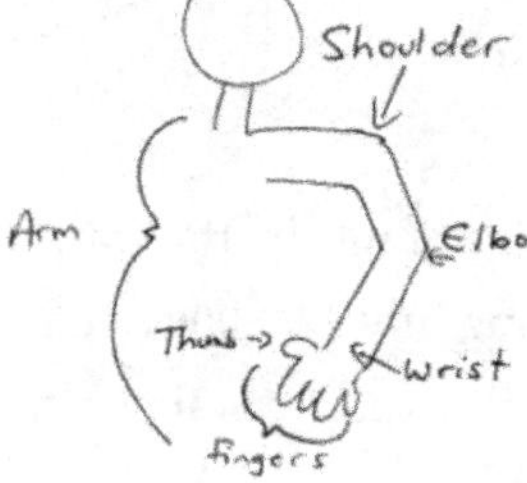

This is not me, by the way.

Starting July 22, 2000, Denise Hong, the PT, did several exercises with me. I would explain what exercises I did here, but my dad's letter is much better at explaining those exercises than me, so here is his letter from August 1, 2000:

Dear Friends of Maureen,

Maureen is now in the Acute Rehabilitation facility at the Davies campus of California Pacific Medical Center. She is in room 3___ in the South Tower. The Davies campus is at Castro and Duboce streets in San Francisco.

From her bed, Maureen has a great view of Eureka Valley, the area that surrounds the Castro. It gets a lot more sun than some other parts of the city, so it is usually quite beautiful to look at. There is a large dining room/lounge area close to Maureen's room. It has the same view of Eureka Valley as well as the South of Market area and the bay. At meal times, it is often filled with families who have brought a complete dinner to share with their father, mother, whatever. In the rehabilitation facility, Maureen wears her normal clothes, so the whole ambiance is much better than a normal hospital.

She is well into a full schedule of therapy. The language is coming little by little, but every day there is improvement. The medical staff wants her to be challenged to develop her language skills. So when she is groping to see if she can say a word that she has in mind, you give her some slack, as they say. If you have studied a foreign language, you know of those times when you cannot remember a particular word. After a while, you try to rephrase your idea into other words, words that you can remember. And then a little while later, you begin to remember the word that you were striving for in the first place. Little by little, your vocabulary builds and you can express yourself better and better. I think something of this kind is starting to happen with Maureen. It should be encouraged. It is the best way to learn.

A few days ago, her physical therapists began trying to teach Maureen to walk again. Judy and I watched her Sunday in the gymnasium (on the lobby level). She has already learned to move comfortably in a wheelchair. She can scoot around using her left foot for propulsion. For the walking session, her (back-up) therapist Paul used a parallel bar apparatus in the gym. He automatically adjusted the height of the bars to hand level. Then Maureen pulled herself out of her wheelchair, something she has already worked on, and stood up. Then he taught her the sequence of left hand forward, weight on left leg, right foot forward, weight on right leg, and finally left leg forward. He explained about how she has to do each step correctly so that she does not develop bad habits, some of which could lead to destruction of the knee or similar dire consequences. It reminded me of those guys on TV showing a good golf stroke. I am not a golfer and so I do not understand all of the fine points. In fact it seems real difficult how they get all of the pieces together in a single smooth swing. Paul is doing the same thing with Maureen, teaching her all of the particulars that when smoothly put together constitute walking. He points out to her that some things that would not seem so important are really the most important of all. When she pulls herself out of her wheelchair and steadies herself, it is the pelvis that she should focus on. He implies that if you get that part right, the rest of the body will go along with it.

Anyway, she walked along with Paul's help about fifteen feet three times. On the second and third tries, I assisted by pushing the wheelchair behind her just in case she might fall backwards. This allowed Paul to focus on what Maureen was doing. In fact, he had to help her with the movement of her right leg. But I felt that this help will diminish as she becomes more and more adept. Her second and third tries were fairly speedy. She did not hesitate overly long after each sequence.

Last night, my sister Mary Ann . . .

(I call her "MaryAnn")

. . . called and said that she and her husband Chuck were visiting Monday in the afternoon, when Maureen was getting physical therapy from her regular therapist (I think her name is Denise). This time, instead of the parallel bars, Maureen was using a cane! And she walked about the same distance three times. Terrific!

Thanks as always to all of you. Maureen is in good spirits. The move to the rehabilitation center was a boon to her. And having a full day's work of therapy each day, leading to a good night's sleep each night, is very beneficial. But I feel that all of the contact with family and especially friends through visits and cards, etc. keep her spirits up so that she can make the most out of what she is doing.

—Jack and Judy Twomey
    (August 1, 2000)

After I had my stroke, I couldn't walk,
but the physical therapists felt that in
time I would be able to walk again.
I needed a brace on my right leg to
walk, but I could do it.

In the wheelchair I did NOT have the brace on my right leg, so if I tried to stand up, I fell. With the brace on, I could walk with a PT there to help me . . . but even with the brace on, I could not walk alone. Not yet . . .

Pictures from Davies Campus, July/August 2000)

In the gym:

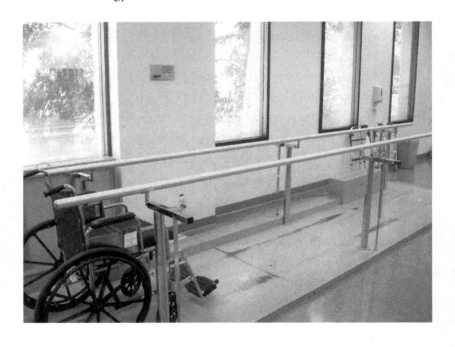

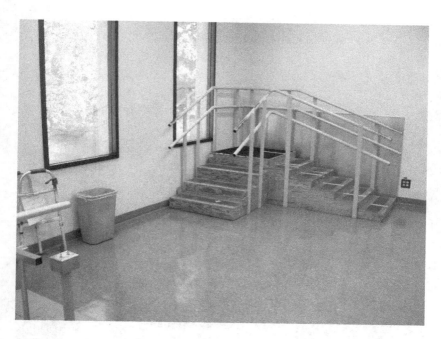

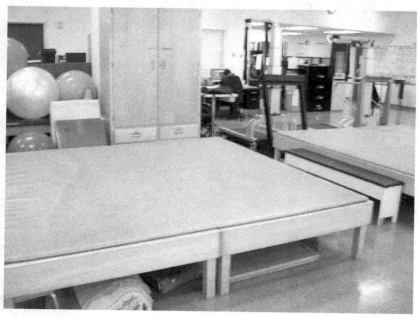

And outside Davies Campus:

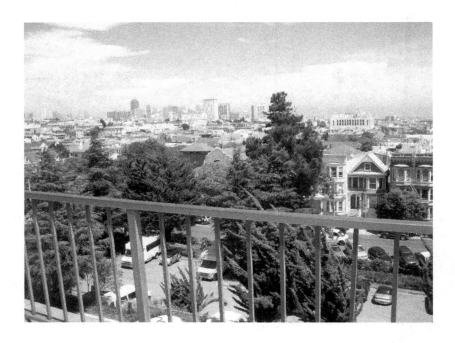

When I was not in PT, OP, or
speech therapy, I practiced re-learning
everything one letter at a time:

bed   and   KEy   W~~~~all

cat   be   Leg   X

well   can   Mom

at   dad   Nat   Yea

milky   end   On   Zoz

no   fig   Pea

bell   Q

dog   get   ~~Rap~~ Ran

tell   High   Saw

wow   In   Tea

    Just   U

        V

I couldn't think of any letter for Q, U, V, or X, and I spelled "zoo" wrong. Darn.

Sometimes I forgot how to spell the word, so I peeked. Like "just"—I think I knew the "ju" part, but I couldn't remember the two other letters, so I peeked at the end of the word to help me finish it.

I remembered the Avon Walk
for Breast Cancer and realized it was
already over (it had happened July 28–
July 30).

Shoot.

(CHAPTER 12)

I was almost done with my second week. They said I was getting better, and I thought so too.

But the beginning of the third week I was kind of getting nervous. Only two weeks left! "Okay," I told myself, "you can do it . . ."

Soon it was going to be four weeks, and I was going to get out. But I still couldn't walk alone. And I could talk, but not a lot . . . :-l

They felt I was still getting better, so they decided to extend my stay at the rehab to five weeks total (July 21–Aug. 21). "Okay, you can do this Maureen!" I told myself.

Then I was *still* improving, so they gave me another week (till August 28).

Everyone who came and visited me
said, "Oh, it's a lovely view." I was
glad to have visitors, but it was more
work for me because I had to appear
happy ("Oh, thank you so much for
coming!"). I knew if I appeared to be
positive more people would come to
visit me.

One day a copywriter from GMO
came to see me, and he gave me one of
the ads I'd written. I still couldn't read
much at all, but I didn't want him to
know that, so I looked at the ad for ten
seconds or so—it might as well have
been written in a foreign language!—
and then said, "Hey—great!"

Studies show

that

hearing loss

AFFECTS

MOSTLY MEN

and

BUGS

MOSTLY WOMEN.

There was a lot of copy in addition to
this page. Maybe my ad was clever, but
I couldn't read the words anymore.
Well, hopefully inTune Hearing
Center liked it!

When I was still working at TBWA\
Chiat\Day, I had three weeks (or
more) of vacation time. So I took three
weeks off (September 8–28) in 1999
and I went to Europe with Rick Steves'
Europe Through the Back Door Tours.
I flew to Amsterdam, where I met
nineteen other people, plus two tour
guides. (Rick Steves was not there . . .
duh.) It was a good group! We went
to the Netherlands, Germany, Austria,
Italy (my favorite), Switzerland, and
France (my second favorite). I had a
fabulous time.

So in November 1999, when I was
freelancing, I sent Rick Steves' ETBD
a cover letter, a resume, and a brief
summary of my travel experience,
including this:

The top 10 reasons (that may not be readily apparent from the attached resumé) why Maureen Twomey would make a wonderful ETBD assistant tour guide:

10. I worked as a UCLA Orientation Counselor for two summers, where every three days I led new groups of freshmen and transfer students on extensive (and, might I say, very entertaining) tours around campus, taught them about academic requirements and university life, helped them enroll in classes, and counseled each student individually. So I have a great deal of experience in leading, teaching and entertaining groups and orientating (is that a word?) them to a new environment. I'm also now quite skilled at memorizing lots of new names.

9. I love Europe.

8. I'm extremely organized and detail-oriented, which I feel would be strong assets for an assistant tour guide. I have a great deal of administrative experience, both full-time (as an account group secretary, an account assistant and a traffic department assistant) and volunteer (I've served as the administrative coordinator for three different organizations). And I'm as happy taking care of these behind-the-scenes details as I am in performing more "in the spotlight" duties.

7. I love to walk and climb stairs. Enough said.

6. I'm currently freelancing, so it would be no trouble for me to take time off in order to assist on tours.

5. I'm adept at picking up the basics (or more) of other languages in order to communicate politely and effectively in foreign countries. I studied French in high school and Italian in college (well, okay, only a quarter's worth, but I'm planning to continue studying Italian this January). And of course I always have my Rick Steves' phrase book in case I ever need to order fish ("just the head, please") or ask "is it free?" in French, Italian or German.

4. I love Europe.

3. I accidentally left my ETBD Travel Clothesline in the hotel in Haarlem, and if I assisted a "Best of Europe" tour, I'd be able to reclaim it. (Of course, I would be happy to assist on any Rick Steves tour, but that *was* a great clothesline.)

2. I'm a gracious, polite, friendly and most importantly, flexible traveler.

1. I love Europe.

Admittedly, that wasn't as knee-slapping funny as a real-live "Top 10 List," but hopefully it's given you a better idea of who I am apart from my current employment as an advertising copywriter...

I copied Rick Steves on the e-mail too.

In January 2000, I found out I didn't get the job. I was disappointed—but thank heavens I wasn't in Europe when I had a stroke.

(Chapter 13)

August 21, 2000

Dad came to visit, and he got me dinner. I wondered what was wrong with him. He told me that Bill, his brother, had died the day before. We were in the rec room. He was crying, and then I was crying.

MaryAnn, Chuck, and my Aunt Marge came the day after. They reassured me that they were terribly distraught about Bill, but they were all right.

They were trying to be very positive. I was trying to explain myself, but I couldn't.

Marge said, "Oh, I FEEL for you!" She took the words right out of my mouth.

Later, after they left, I still was so sad. "Uncle Bill was so healthy—so fit," I thought. "Now he is in heaven, and that is wonderful; but his wife, Aunt Gay, Terri, Willie, and all of us are so sad.

"Lord, you should have taken me instead . . . After all, I'm so, so sick still. But Bill has so much left to give! Why did you take him first? It should have been me," I thought.

Some time later, I thought again about what Anne Lamott said in *Bird by Bird*: To be a good writer you have to write it all down right away. If you don't write it down—you forget about it.

Now that I'd had the stroke, I had so many things to talk about—but I couldn barely speak, so I couldn't say to another person in the room, "Hey, write this down."

It was so frustrating that I had done creative writing before but now I couldn't. So many people could write easily, but I couldn't.

I think all I was wondering was, "What am I good at?" I couldn't think of anything I was good at now. My family and friends were praying for me, and the medical people were wishing me good thoughts too. I guessed I was somewhat better. But now what was I good at . . . anything??

Some afternoon, two women came to visit me, Patricia and Ellen. They had both had strokes (I'm not sure when, but they seemed fine), and now they were volunteering for "Stroke Survivors Starting Over."

Then wanted to know if I had any questions for them. I couldn't think of any; but even if I could have, I mostly couldn't talk, and no one was there to help me.

They gave me a pamphlet—

"San Freawftfeg Steks Recbeeceh Direhsto," I read—and they gave me their cards.

I can't remember who came in next (family, staff, etc.), but when they did, I said something like "What's that say?" (I was asking about the pamphlet.)

"San Francisco Stroke Resource Directory," they read.

"Ohhhh . . ." I said.

He/she read me some stuff from

inside the pamphlet, but I was tired so I told him/her I'd read it later (or rather, someone else would).

:-1

❀   ❀   ❀

There was a woman in rehab who was the same age or so as me. She hadn't had a stroke, but she was going through something difficult too. I didn't get a chance to talk to her. Soon she was so much better and was going home. She thanked everyone, and she was so happy.

When I overheard her thanking everyone, I thought, "I am really happy for her!" But at the same time I thought, "Why am I not better too?"

❀   ❀   ❀

When I first got to rehab, I thought, "I'll be so much better soon." After six or so weeks there, everyone said I was better, but I was the one living with me every day, and I'd thought I would be much better by now than I was. I thought I would be making much more progress—walking alone, walking faster every day.

Every day, I worked with a reading instructor. But it was so basic. For instance, they had several objects—a pen, a heart, a frog, a watch, etc.—and I was supposed to identify them. In the beginning, I couldn't think of the word. It was truly so frustrating. I was a copywriter—words were supposed to be my thing—and I was stuck with "What's that object? Oh, it's a frog!" Why was it so difficult?

They held a speech lesson for us, and most of the people there were in their sixties to seventies. I was thirty-three! I was thinking in my head, "Everyone is doing so much better than me."

The worst part was when during an activity—speech lessons or whatever—the other people would introduce themselves: "Hi, I'm Martha." "My name is Fred."

I could do my name, but sometimes I forgot it completely. Maureen or Twomey . . . I couldn't remember at all. AAAAAAAAAAAAAAAH!!! It was so embarrassing that everyone else was so much more accomplished than me. I thought after six weeks of work,

I should be much, much, much more improved.

At times I would cry and not know for sure what I was crying for.

When I was inside the rehab building, I felt safe to cry.

Outside there was a view; you could see downtown and the Bay Bridge. It was quite glorious. I didn't cry when I was looking at that view.

"Hmmmmm . . ." I thought. "Maybe I should move my bed outside; it's a great view, and then maybe I'll never cry."

Inside again, I didn't have to worry about people looking at me when I cried. "Am I never going to be 100 percent better? Is it always going to be this way? Did I do something wrong? Could I have done anything different?"

"Oh wait—sometimes I get irritated or upset with things or people," I thought, "but usually I apologize after. But is God mad at me? Is he so mad at me that he did this to spite me?"

Then, all of a sudden, I felt God in my presence, and I remembered a dream I'd had in January of that year.

Remember the dream you had

in January? said the Lord. (I knew He was not talking out loud, but I could hear Him as plain as day.) *You know, the dream about being stuck underwater?*

(I was under the water. I was stuck under a rock, so I couldn't get myself up to the surface. I was drowning and I couldn't do anything about it. I was dying. Then, suddenly, I could BREATHE, even though I was still UNDERWATER! It was amazing! I realized that I was going to heaven— and then suddenly I woke up. It was only a dream, but it was so real!)

I wanted you to remember the dream, said the Lord.

> "'I know what I am planning for you,' declares the Lord. 'I have good plans for you, not plans to hurt you. I will give you hope and a good future.'"
> —Jeremiah, 29:11

God said, *I will be there for you every step of the way. But I'm not ready for you to go to heaven yet. Your family and friends will be there for you. And I love you, Maureen.*

I was still crying, but now I was crying out of hope.

(Thankfully, I didn't have mascara on my eyes; it would have been a mess.)

;)

and

AFTER . . .

THE END.

Oh, wait a minute! There's more to tell you . . .

and

AFTER . . .

(CHAPTER 14)

The next day I was sitting having
lunch in the rec room. Two women—
they were about sixty or seventy I
think—were in there having lunch
as well. They had both had strokes
too, but I think only minor ones;
their speech was fine. They both had
wheelchairs too, but they could walk.

One of the women (I think her
name was Lillian) said to me, "You are
so pretty!"

"Are you talking to me?!" I
thought. I had a helmet on because
some of my skull was missing, and
there were many other things wrong
with me, too. Maybe she was wearing
an old pair of glasses (i.e., she couldn't
really see me).

But she *was* looking at me, and she truly meant it—and yes, I think she could see fine.

"That's so nice," I thought. "Maybe I should tip her?"

;)

❀   ❀   ❀

"CALIFORNIA PACIFIC MEDICAL – DAVIES CAMPUS . . . LOCOMOTION:

WALKING AND STAIR TAKING: THE PATIENT IS **TOTALLY DEPENDENT . . ."**

I still couldn't walk alone. Not even with a brace on my right leg.

On Sunday, September 3, I was exercising with Susan (another PT person). I had a belt on me so she could help to hold me up.

We were outside, and I was walking ahead of her. Then all of a sudden—"Wait . . . am I walking without you?" I asked.

Susan hadn't told me because she didn't want to interfere—but yes, I was walking all on my own! "Oh my gosh!" I thought. "I can walk alone!"

Update:

"CALIFORNIA PACIFIC MEDICAL – DAVIES CAMPUS . . .
LOCOMOTION:

WALKING AND STAIR TAKING: THE PATIENT IS
MAXIMAL."

. . . But not "TOTALLY DEPENDENT." Whoohoooo!

(Note: No, I'm NOT saying that if you just pray enough you will walk again. Everyone has a different situation.

I'm just telling my story.)

Thursday, August 31, 2000, they had given me goals for Week 7. The ending was in pink pen . . . BUT on September 3, I finally walked, so they added a new goal in black:

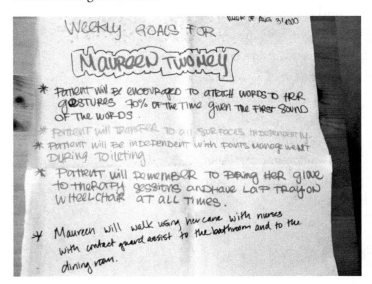

WHOOHOOOOO!

❀   ❀   ❀

The San Francisco Prosthetic Orthotic
Service (S.F. POS) specializes in
individual, customized orthopedic
and prosthetic appliances. They came
to Davies Campus every Tuesday. Now
two of the guys, Chris Chandler and
Wayne Koniuk, were going to do my
new right leg brace.

Michael Plafker from S.F. POS
wrote the following about my brace:

> "AFO" ankle foot orthosis –
> Helps clear toes when swinging through
> Helps reduce knee hyperextension when standing
> (custom made)

Score!

❀   ❀   ❀

Really hard work . . . well, for me,
anyway:

SELECT THE WORD THAT NAMES EACH PICTURE 100% 09/05

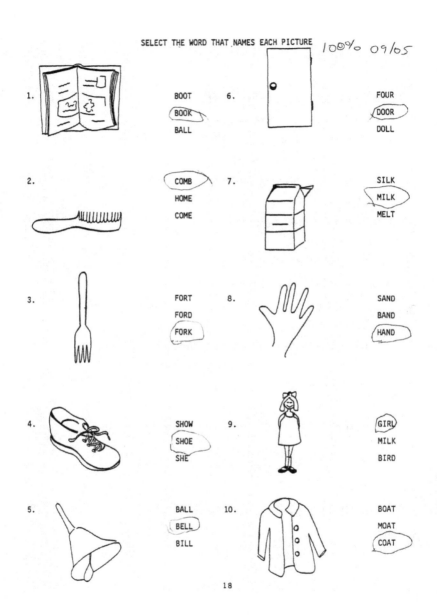

1. BOOT
   BOOK
   BALL

2. COMB
   HOME
   COME

3. FORT
   FORD
   FORK

4. SHOW
   SHOE
   SHE

5. BALL
   BELL
   BILL

6. FOUR
   DOOR
   DOLL

7. SILK
   MILK
   MELT

8. SAND
   BAND
   HAND

9. GIRL
   MILK
   BIRD

10. BOAT
    MOAT
    COAT

18

154   Before, Afdre, and After

COPYING WORDS: Picture Identification — Noun Choice

1. Is this a rose or a cake?

It is a __CAKE cake__

). Is this a shirt or a table?

It is a __table table__

1. Is this a ball or a truck?

It is a __ball ball__

2. Is this a cat or a fish?

It is a __fish fish__

3. Is this a window or a hose?

It is a __window window__

14. Is this a hand or a toe?

It is a __hand hand__

15. Is this a door or a tree?

It is a __tree tree__

16. Is this a book or a coat?

It is a __book book__

17. Is this a man or a shoe?

It is a __man man__

18. Is this a flower or a tree?

It is a __flower flower__

19. Is this a knife or a spoon?

It is a __spoon spoon__

I think I wrote the words twice ("cake cake," "table table," etc.) because I thought I would learn it faster that way than if I only did it once.

(Chapter 15)

"When I leave rehab," I wondered, "where will I go? There is no other rehab facility close by—they're all booked. The closest one is two hours away. And everyone else (my family and friends) works full-time at their jobs.

Sometime after that, MaryAnn and Chuck said, "We would be happy to have you stay with us." They had recently retired (and remember, MaryAnn was a nurse!). They also lived in San Francisco and they had a huge home. Their address is: (kidding; I'm not going to tell you . . . sorry).

Thank you, MaryAnn and Chuck!!!

September 7, 2000

Goals for Week 8:

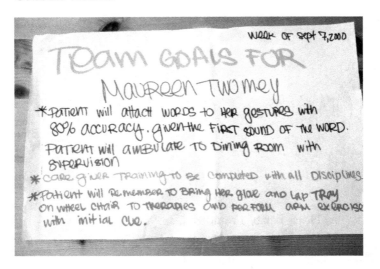

Week of Sept 7, 2000

Team Goals for Maureen Twomey

*Patient will attach words to her gestures with 80% accuracy. given the first sound of the word. Patient will ambulate to Dining Room with supervision

*care giver training to be completed with all disciplines

*Patient will remember to bring her glove and lap tray on wheel chair to therapies and perform arm exercise with initial cue.

I had six other goal sheets, for Weeks 1 to 6, but I don't have them. Maybe other people stole them and have them framed on their wall?

William Johnson and Sherri (Sherri lived across the hall from William) came to see me, and they brought Salinger, my cat). She was soooo scared—I think she thought, "WHY AM I IN THE HOSPITAL?!" (Then again, maybe she wasn't thinking about that. Anyway . . .)

I wondered if Salinger even recognized me. Now I had a helmet on my head, and she hadn't seen me since June 6—now it was September 11. But William put her on my lap, and she immediately calmed down.

"See? She knows you! . . . Maureen, you look great! So much better now!"

It was so good to see them, AND Salinger, but I wasn't ready to have Salinger come with me to MaryAnn and Chuck's house yet.

"Don't worry about your cat," William said. "Take as long as you want. When you get better, Salinger will come home with you."

Man, I was so grateful!

At the Davies rehab, when you are close to going home, they take you off campus to see how you adjust. Around September 12, Joanie and Kalynn and I went to a coffee shop just two or so blocks from the hospital. I went in my wheelchair because:

1) Outside of the Davies campus, there are a lot of medium and steep hills. I

always had a brace on my leg now, but it would be better for me to practice on level streets at first. So Joanie pushed me in the wheelchair (thanks, Joanie).

2) I only could walk a short block on my own at this point, so it was nice to have the wheelchair so I could sit back down when I needed to rest.

We went inside the coffee place. I thought the guy who worked there would say, "Wow what's that on your head!?"

Well, he didn't. Now that I think about that, though, the coffee shop is really close to Davies campus, so I guess they see tons of people who work or live there. They're probably used to it.

Good mocha, by the way.

When the new brace was ready, Chris Chandler and Wayne Koniuk came back to have me try it out. It was a half-leg brace. They wanted to see me walk around a bit and make sure my brace was working well, so I tried it on and walked around a little, back and forth. They said the right leg was "locking back," so they would get me some knee support to wear with the brace. It was called a "Swedish Knee Cage."

"Oooooh Swedish!" I said. I was going to say something after that, like, "Do I have to talk with an accent when I have it on?"

It was a simple joke, but I couldn't get the words out of my mouth. Shoot.

(In hindsight, it's not that funny. So there was another thing I wasn't good at anymore.)

September 13, 2000
I was still in rehab, but it was almost time for me to go home with Chuck and MaryAnn. Chuck, MaryAnn, and Dad were there for my going-away party. The rehab people gave me a cake, and then we went to lunch at a restaurant. I guess they liked me. ;)

Later, when I got back to my room, I got scared. I thought, "I should stay here." Three and a half months had passed since my stroke now, and I'd thought that after six weeks in the hospital and eight weeks in rehab, I'd be 100 percent better— but I wasn't. My OP and PT were telling me I was ready to go home, but I still needed someone to walk close behind me when I walked or I'd fall. "I'm not ready!" I thought.

I'd also thought that after eight weeks I'd be much closer to reading fully. I was doing better, but I still couldn't even read a full sentence. "Am I doing something wrong?" I thought. "Can I stay? I'm scared to leave."

Well . . .

CALIFORNIA PACIFIC MEDICAL – DAVIES CAMPUS,
TWOMEY, MAUREEN E ... ADMIT: 07/24/00
DISCHARGE: 9/14/00
DISCHARGE REHABILITATION SUMMARY

DISCHARGE DIAGNOSES . . .

DISCHARGE FUNCTIONS REHABILITATION STATUS:
SELF-CARE:
EATING: THE PATIENT IS MINIMAL ASSIST.
GROOMING: THE PATIENT IS MINIMAL ASSIST.
BATHING: THE PATIENT IS MODERATE ASSIST.

DRESSING BODY: THE PATIENT IS MINIMAL/MODERATE ASSIST.

TRANSFERS:

BED, CHAIR, WHEELCHAIR, BED AND SHOWER TRANSFERS: THE PATIENT IS MODERATE ASSIST.

LOCOMOTION:

WALKING AND STAIR TAKING: THE PATIENT IS MAXIMAL.

COMMUNICATION:

COMPREHENS: THE PATIENT IS MODERATE ASSIST.
EXPRESSION: THE PATIENT IS MAXIMAL ASSISTANCE

SOCIAL COGNITION:

SOCIAL INTERACTION: THE PATIENT IS MINIMAL ASSIST.
PROBLEM SOLVING: THE PATIENT IS MODERATE ASSIST.
MEMORY: THE PATIENT IS MODERATE ASSIST.

—STEPHEN NG, M.D.

(Chapter 16)

September 14, 2000

So I went home with MaryAnn and
Chuck. Once I got there, I mostly
stayed in the cushy chair in the family
room. When I wanted to get up, I had
to first get my helmet on. I had a new
cane so I could balance myself, but
someone still had to stay near me in
case I fell.

The beds were upstairs. There
were stairs on both sides, so I thought
I was going to be able to do it myself.
But Chuck and MaryAnn were helping
me up and down the stairs in case I
fell at the beginning. So when I was
downstairs in the family room, and
I wanted to rest, I didn't say, "Hey
MaryAnn and Chuck! I'm tired; help

me upstairs again to my bedroom. Then, when I'm done napping, help me down again." (What am I, the Queen?)

No, if I wanted to rest, I just went to the living room. Soon I was able to go walk fully on my own and didn't even have to use a cane inside.

When I first came home and was struggling for words, I thought everyone would be impatient with me because I couldn't get the words out of my mouth—I couldn't explain myself. Some people would have been rushing me and pushing me or trying to speak for me. But my family and friends always told me to take my time. My dad once said, "We're not silent because we're irritated, we're silent because we want to hear what you have to say. Take your time."

All of a sudden I could express myself better.

Of course, soon after that, some people stopped by. When I sat down, I took my helmet off. Most of the people who were there kept looking at me when I was talking, but some other people seemed like they didn't want to look at me. I thought at first, "Are they mad at me? Did I say something wrong?"

After they left, I realized I
probably should have kept my helmet
on. Whoops.

❀   ❀   ❀

(MaryAnn took some notes tracking
my progress)

9/14/00

First day home—Spoke on the phone with Suzanne, and
was able to communicate better. Later spoke with her Aunt
Marge, repeated her name, and said that she was going to
come back 100%.

Had dinner with her father (Jack) & Judy, and Suzanne.
Evening went very well.

Did well on stairs . . .

(etc.)

9/15/00

Sat up @ 9 am – Some assistance entering the shower.

(There was a handicap chair
already inside the shower, but at first it
was difficult to get in.)

Dressed with very little assistance. Came downstairs with
Chuck supervising her. Met the visiting physical therapist.
She interviewed Maureen and did some physical assess-
ments. Walked around the house for 5 or 10 minutes (with
one of us behind her, but she was walking well). Occasion-

ally, she was not putting enough weight on her right leg though.

Her appetite is very good.

She described her trip to Europe last year and needed some prompting to correct opening of the Olympics.

Slept well . . .

PT (Joyce), OP (Barbara), and Speech (Alan) would come to my home (well, MaryAnn and Chuck's home), three times a week.

The first day I saw Joyce, my physical therapist, she took these notes:

ALL PURPOSE HOME PROGRAM SHEET

PATIENT'S NAME LAST	PATIENT'S NO.	DATE	TIME A M	P M
Twomey, Maureen		9		

Seated

TRUNK Rotation - Twisting
Independent   10 x

TRUNK - Foward + Back
                10 x

Side BENDING
                10 x

STANDING

assist · Walking · Back walking
                Front walking
                Side Stepping
                (Chair Behind)

assist · TRUNK Rotation · Twisting
· Side Bend   5 Resis.
· Hip Rotation
· Standing by Chair
· STANDING at SINK

STAFF SIGNATURE

❀ ❀ ❀

MaryAnn's notes about my progress
again:

9/16/00

Up at 9:00 am . . . Did much better in the shower chair (getting in) . . .

Dressed without assistance.

Walked around the house for 6 times + 10 minutes . . .

Visited with her brother (Mike & Joan), who live some distances away. They had not seen her in some time (but they talk on the photo regularly). Delighted with her progress . . .

Later, my cousin Kathy Looney and a guy she was dating at the time stopped by. Chuck and MaryAnn were cooking in the kitchen.

Kathy and her date and I were sitting around the dinner table. He was talking and talking and talking. (Granted, some people talk more then other people. And when they're talking about interesting topics, it's fine. Not this time.)

Kathy got up and went to the kitchen to see if she could do anything for Chuck and MaryAnn. The boyfriend was still seated with me. But now he couldn't think of anything to say. So I spoke up, trying to get my words out, but he quickly got up and went to the kitchen.

Oh my God! I was talking, but

instead of listening to me he just walked out of the room. "Hey," I thought, "I know you can hear me talking. At least say 'Excuse me'!" I even had my helmet on, so I didn't look scary. He was so rude! ("Well," I thought, "when he was talking, *he* was totally stuck on himself. So I couldn't care less if he speaks to me or not.")

When we all sat down for dinner, he started talking again; not about anything interesting, just him, him, him: "BLAB, BLAB, BLAB, BLAB, BLAB, BLAB, BLAB, BLAB, BLAB, BLAB, BLAB, BLAB, BLAB, BLAB . . ." Maybe two or three months later, Kathy broke up with him, and everyone said, "Thank God!" and "I didn't like him either."

More notes MaryAnn wrote down:

9/17/00
. . . Dressed herself with no assistance.

9/18/00
Nurse visited, did physical assessment, vital signs, etc.
Barbara, the OP, visited—did an assessment and some exercises on Maureen's right arm.

Then she gave me more arm
exercises to do.

Joyce, the PT, came at 1:30 pm. She gave Maureen a lot of
exercises.
They were exercises to help relearn of neuron pathways.
Maureen seemed very happy with the workout.

I started working with Alan, my
reading/writing person, and my
penmanship started to get much
better even though I was writing with
the wrong hand. So I think my writing
was neater than Alan's now . . . no,
really. The first part is Alan's notes:

Write ~~for~~ 15 sentences per
day. First 2 days some/a, <u>then</u>
~~those/that~~ .

I want (some
a
_____
~~these~~ those
that) _____ object.

1. I want some beer.
2. I want some wine.
3. I want some cows.
4. I want a milk.
5. I want some tea.
6. I want some coffee.
7. I want some onion.
8. I want some orange.
9. I want a banana.
10. I want some broccoli.
11. I want some lettuce.
12. I want some bean.
13. I want some grape.
14. I want some chicken
15. I want some liver.

"Broccoli and liver," I said. "I hate
broccoli and liver!!!"

Alan also gave me face exercises
to do:

ALL PURPOSE HOME PROGRAM SHEET

PATIENT'S NAME LAST Twomey	FIRST Maureen	PATIENT'S NO. 09477	DATE 9/20/01	TIME A.M. P.M.

1) Lick lips all around with tongue tip. 10 clockwise 10 counter clockwise.

2) Say /oo ee   oo ee   oo ee/

   /Ah oh   Ah oh   Ah oh/

   Do 10 sets count between.

3) Push tongue into cheek R → L
   x10.

4) Lick "outside" of teeth with lips closed. Keep lips closed.

5) Take vowels
   A E I O U. ou ai
         oh (you)   (hay)
   put them in series of 3.   x10
         "   4   x5.

   2 x / day.

STAFF SIGNATURE

Alan Grant MS-SLP.

What? I don't remember that I had
a problem with my face/lip/tongue.
Did everyone else notice? D'oh!

❀ ❀ ❀

Someone told me, "You have lost some of your brain tissue. But the brain has so, so much that it will find another way to allow you to read and write again."

I didn't realize how much practice it would take. I thought, "I can't write in sentences yet, but in time, I will gradually get better." I was determined to do everything, but I also had to rest a lot. I reminded myself that nothing was going to change overnight.

"Okay," I thought.

One night we decided to go out to dinner. The restaurant was only fourteen blocks away from MaryAnn and Chuck's house, so I thought we would walk there and then walk back when we were done. (That's twenty-eight blocks total, but you already know how to add.)

"Maureen," MaryAnn said, "can you really walk fourteen blocks there and fourteen blocks home?"

"Oh . . . no," I said. The furthest I had gone was two blocks (one block and back). So we drove instead.

"Maybe next week I'll be 100 percent better," I thought . . . haaaa.

❀ ❀ ❀

I still had part of my skull missing on the left side of my head, so I hadn't gone to the hair salon for four months. Dad suggested that I go to the salon and get my hair trimmed.

"Uhhhh?!" I thought. I had to wait for the surgery when they would put back my skull, and *then* I could go to the salon. In the meantime, though, I had one side long and one side really short. (Also, now everyone could tell I had many gray hairs . . . yes, I started turning gray when I was only twenty-two years old! So usually someone colored my hair every so often, but I hadn't had that done since my stroke, either.)

In fact, my swelling had completely gone down (I thought). "I can have my surgery now, and THEN get my hair done," I said. "Well, not NOW, but I can at least make my appointment to have my surgery done."

But my dad said the doctor still didn't think I was ready.

(WHAT?!)

Dad said the doctor said maybe October or later.

AAAAAAAAHHHH!

I didn't want to go to a salon because I was afraid to shock people with my missing skull (you're reading the book right now and you're thinking the same thing too!). But my dad talked me into going to a salon in Noe Valley, a neighborhood in San Francisco. It was a small place: there were only two other stylists besides the person who was going to cut my hair.

There were other people in the shop, and I was sure they were thinking, "Oh my gosh!" I wanted to say, "I'm sorry," but I couldn't get the words out.

The lady who cut my hair was very nice, though, and she did the best that she could do with my hair.

More work. (Thanks, Alan, for the somewhat better penmanship.)

Hand tap c̄ phrases   9/28/00

Do you know them?

What is your name?

I want some more

That is too much

Did you like that.?

Where are you going?

Why did they go?

Is it time yet?

When will he come here?

Why don't you take one?

What did you say?

I don't know them.

Isn't it too bad.

Take your time.

DATE	NAME
10-6-00	Maureen, you are truly a goddess! Your self dedication is so evident — Keep up the great work!
10-7-00	Maureen, you look better each time I see you! I love the short hair! Love, Stephanie
10-8-00	Maureen— we're so thrilled to see you. You look fabulous. Love, Jnfn
10-9-00	M· I CANNOT BELIEVE YOU'RE PROGRESS YOU LOOK FABULOUS + I'M SO GLAD TO SEE YOU. JENN

Now YOU sign it:

DATE	NAME
	Hi Maureen,

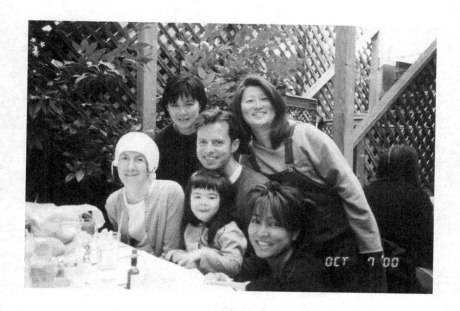

Can you tell which one I am?

(Top: Karen Avery, John Avery, Riki Komachi; Sitting down: Me and my helmet, Sydney A., Jenn Muranaka-Chaney)

Chuck never took pictures until my skull was back intact . . . I don't know why. Haaaa.

(Chapter 17)

Well finally, on October 20, or so,
I went back to the hospital to have
the operation to put my skull back
together. But first I had to shave my
head. (Well, *I* didn't have to do it;
someone else did it.) Mmmmmm .
. . Maybe whoever did it was a real
hair stylist? In that case I should
have gotten his card, in case I need a
haircut like that again.

Anyway, now I was bald! "Bad
hair look for me," I thought; but when
the operation was done, I wouldn't
have to wear the helmet EVER again,
so I wasn't too upset!

Actually, I didn't have to shave
ALL of my hair off, just the part of my
head that the doctors had to work on
(the left side). So some people thought
it would be fine to keep the hair on

my right side intact. But I thought, "Why?" Maybe other people who have brain surgery keep their hair. Not me—I'll just wear hats.

So, to the operation!

It was a success! (Well I was asleep, but they told me after that it was all back intact.)

But when I was still in the operation room, I started to wake up and I had a seizure . . .

W h a t ' s ~ h a p p e n i n g ~ t~o m~e ~ ? W~h~y ~ i~s ~ m~y ~ b~o~d~y t~u~r~n~I~n~g l~e~f~t~? P~l~e~a~s~e h~e~l~p m~e ~ ! M~~a~~k~~e i~~t s~~t~~o~~p~~!~~ ! M~~a~~k~~e i~~t s~~t~~o~~p~~!~~ ! M~~a~~k~~e i~~t s~~t~~o~~p~~!~~! M~~a~~k~~e i~~t s~~t~~o~~p~~!~~! M~~a~~k~~e i~~t s~~t~~o~~p~~!~~ ! M~~a~~k~~e i~~t s~~t~~o~~p~~!~~! M~~a~~k~~e i~~t s~~t~~o~~p~~!~~! M~~a~~k~~e i~~t s~~t~~o~~p~~!~~! . . .

I thought I was having a terrible nightmare again. But it was real. AAAAAAAAAAAAH!

Eventually it stopped. MAN. The doctor gave me Dilantin, which is a generic, very inexpensive drug for treating seizures, but it turned out that I have a BIG allergic reaction to Dilantin. I didn't take it again. The doctor thought the seizure was a one-time thing, so rather then having me try another brand of seizure pill, he didn't prescribe me anything.

Anyway, when I woke up I was in bed and my head was turned to the right, resting on the pillow.

Now that the operation was done and my head was fully healed, I thought, "Oh my gosh, maybe my brain is intact now and I can see on my right side again!"

So I slowly took my head off the pillow: "Oh my gosh! I can see all the way to the right side! My sight is back to normal! Whoohooo!"

Oh wait . . . nevermind. :-l

(If you want to know what it's like for me, look straight ahead, and hold up a pencil in front of your face. Move it slowly to the right. For me, all of sudden it disappears. Shoot.)

So, was I 100 percent better now? (Was I smart again?) When I woke up and my head was back together, I thought at first, "Maybe now that everything is back together, I'll be able to read and write again.

Well, I guess my brain said, "No Maureen, it's not going to happen today."

"Shoot again," I said.

"Okay," I thought, "maybe tomorrow when I wake up, I'll be reading and writing again. I've gone through so much. Now maybe God will say, "I'll put your reading and writing instantly back to normal."

Still waiting . . .

Later, when I was still at the hospital at CPMC, the anesthesiologist who had helped with my operation came to see me. It was so nice that he was concerned about my seizure.

"Hey, wait a minute," I thought, "is he hitting on me?" (Then I thought, "Yeah, right.")

My skull was FINALLY back to normal! "Now everyone can look at me and they won't be able to tell anything is wrong," I thought.

I would just have to wear a hat until my hair came back. (Stephanie,

Riki, Jenn, Mari, and other people
who gave me hats . . . thank you!)

After the surgery, some people
still couldn't look at me, though.
Hmmmmm . . . maybe they just didn't
like hats?

(Chapter 18)

I thought I would return back to work
in October, because I thought I still
had a job at GMO. ("Right, Maureen,"
I thought after.) But I had much
more to relearn again. So I returned
to Davies Campus, now as an out-
patient, three times a week.

Some of the arm exercises I had
to do:

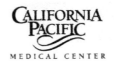

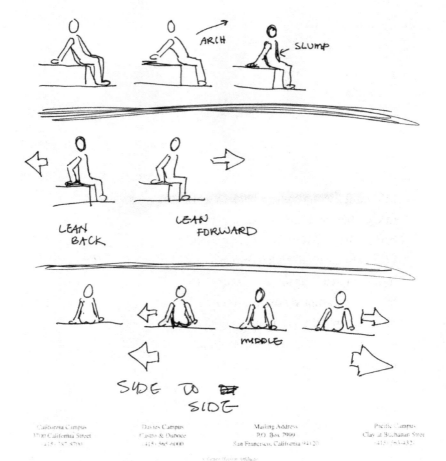

California Campus
3700 California Street

Davies Campus
Castro & Duboce

Mailing Address
P.O. Box 7999
San Francisco, California 94120

Pacific Campus
Clay at Buchanan Street

And leg exercises (this is later, in 2001, but it's the same things I did in 2000):

CALIFORNIA PACIFIC

MEDICAL CENTER

6/7/01

1. Lie on your back, knees bent
   Lift your hips
   lift left foot up & down

2. Mini knee bends standing - without the brace; shoes on

3. Stand tall scoot left foot out & in

4. Try to move your right leg forward as if it is on a line during walking

Sonya Richardson

California Campus
3700 California Street
(415) 387-8700

Davies Campus
Castro & Duboce
(415) 565-6000

Mailing Address
P.O. Box 7999
San Francisco, California 94120

Pacific Campus
Clay at Buchanan Street
(415) 563-4321

A Sutter Health Affiliate

When I was at home, I would sit at the table, take off my brace, and do more exercises.

Deborah Van Atta was now my

speech, reading, and writing person. Here is what she wrote:

California Pacific Medical Center
Outpatient Department

SPEECH/LANGUAGE PROGRESS REPORT FOR THER-
APY EXTENSION

PATIENT NAME: Maureen Twomey
DATE: 11/28/00

THERAPIST: Deborah Van Atta, MS CCC-SLP

EVALUATION FINDINGS:
33 years woman admitted to CPMC initially 6/7/00 with massive acute left hemisphere infarct of the left occipital-temporal-posterior parietal lobe with s/p left temporal craniotomy and partial temporal lobectomy. Left PCA and MCA infarct secondary to left carotid dissection with anomalous fetal PCA circulation. PMH: No significant history reported. Following medical stabilization, pt transferred to Acute Rehab at the Davies Campus on 7/21/00 for speech/language and dysphagia intervention from which she was discharged home 9/14/00 with follow up Home Health.

RESULTS OF EVALUATION ARE AS FOLLOWS:
Expressive: Pt presents with a moderately severe aphasia for verbalizing needs, opinions, etc., although she successfully augments her communication with gestures. Her language errors are characterized by paraphasias, with "empty"

speech largely devoid of content words, e.g. Description of ADP Grocery Store picture: "baby . . . (gesture fall), not sis(ter) . . . (gesture looking)." Re: her language goals, pt stated "I want 100%." Writing: Pt is able to write her name legibly with her unaffected hand. To be further assessed.

COMPREHENSION:

Moderately severe deficits for moderate to complex information. Pt able to follow basic 2 unit body part commands: 90% for primary (e.g. nose), 50% for secondary (e.g. elbow). Her accuracy significantly declines with left/right discrimination imposed, though she is able to spatially distinguish the two. Pt can follow simple directions. Reading: Pt was described as prolific reader before her stroke, but is unable to read at baseline at present due to language, processing, and visual deficits.

COGNITION:

To be further assessed. Pt reportedly has memory deficits second to temporal lobectomy.

PLAN OF TREATMENT:

By 3/30/01 pt will be able to:

1. Access Daily Communicator to express needs, e.g. food choices for meals/marketing list, prioritizing clothing needs, arranging day trips, etc. with 70% accuracy;
2. Name objects in environment 90%, and describe function 70%;
3. Read at word/short phrase level with 80% accuracy;
4. Write names of functional objects with 80% accuracy;
5. Write, recall basic information in organizer 70%.

NUMBER/FREQUENCY/DURATION OF VISITS EXPECTED:

2 x week x 8 weeks, plus 1 x week aphasia group (optional; pending discussion with pt.)

EXPECTED OUTCOME/GOALS:

Pt will maximize her rehabilitation potential for expression, reception, reading, and writing for basic communication within a familiar environment, utilizing augmentation as needed. Electronic AAC aids to be investigated.

—Deborah Van Atta, MS

Gradually, I could read more words but still no full sentences. So Deborah suggested this:

DAILY COMMUNICATOR

For Every Communication Situation

This book has been designed for use by the person with limited verbal skills who retains an ability to read at the word level. It is meant to be used in everyday communication situations. The book is organized into categories commonly encountered in daily life. Not all situations or words needed are listed here. Please feel free to "personalize" this book to fit the user. If something is needed, add it. If something is never used or wanted, cross it out. Change, modify, but above all, encourage daily use of this book as a communication aid to assist the user to become an independent, functional communicator.

(Created By Cynthia Jones, MA CCC/S, Janis Lorman, MA CCC/S) http://www.alimed.com/daily-communicator.html

Here's one page:

Buy/Pay	Forget
Clean	Give/Take
Cook	Go/Stop
Cry	Hear/Listen
Drink	Help
Drive	Hurt
Eat	Kiss
Exercise	Laugh
Explain	Like/Love
Fall/Drop	Make
Fight	Mow
Fill	On/Off
Find/Lose	Open/Close

Action Words

Some other pages:

Basic Needs (Pain, Nurse, Shower . . .)
Feelings (Hungry, Sleepy, Bored . . .)
Men's Clothing (Belt, Hat, Shoes . . .)
Men's Needs (Comb, Deodorant, Razor . . .)
Women's Clothing (Blouse, Coat, Earrings . . .)
Women's Needs (Blush, Lipstick, Curlers . . .) (Haaa)
Meal Needs (Coffee, Coffee, Coffee . . .) (Haaa again)
Places (Airport, Hairdresser, Mall/Store . . .)
Time (Morning, Evening, Minute . . .)
Days (Monday, Friday, Week . . .)
Months/Seasons (May, July, Summer . . .)
Money Matters (Penny, Twenty, Charge . . .)
Weather (Hot, Fog, Hurricane . . .)
Occasions/Holidays (Wedding, St. Patrick's Day, Maureen's Birthday . . .)

Well, it didn't say "Maureen's," but you get the idea . . .

There are many other interactive therapeutic tools located here: http://www.alimed.com/interactive-therapeutics/default.aspx

Between 1993 and 1998 I always made creative cards to send my friends for Christmas. In 1999, I was moving to San Francisco in January and was too

busy to think of a witty Christmas card, so I just bought cards at a gift store and wrote something like, "Sorry . . . I will create a wittier card next year!"

Well, now I had a small (yeah, right) medical problem so in 2000 I bought a card off the rack again at Christmastime and simply wrote, "Love, Maureen ☺."

(Sorry, Morgan Rumpf . . . I remember that voicemail from July, "I look forward to your Christmas card every year, and I want it to be especially creative this year!" Next year, Morgan.)

Anyway, my printing now is much better (and smaller), but in 2000, it was still not very good.

I had forgotten to tell some people that I'd had a stroke, and Trish Cook Borrmann (my high school friend) hadn't seen me in seven months or so. I sent her and Gary a card, and the signature was like a kid's. She thought it was a joke at first.

Whoops. (Now she knows the truth, of course.)

Chuck and MaryAnn always had a Christmas party, and that year was no exception. I invited a couple friends, including Suzanne, a friend of mine who lived in North Beach (S.F.), but had just bought a house in the East Bay. She was going to move in January.

"That's great!" I said. "Hey, can I take your apartment when you move to your new home? I love North Beach!"

"Haaaaa," I thought after . . . Suzanne's place was the same type of building where I use to live—i.e., no elevator. But even if it had had an elevator, I was not ready to do many things by myself.

Thankfully, Chuck was listening to our conversation, and he kindly said something like, "Well, not right now I think."

December 2000
Dear Friends of Maureen,

Hi, not even a hint of bad news this time. Ever since Maureen's final operation, things have been getting back to normal. There has been no recurrence of a seizure, as happened in recovery after replacement of the bone flap. Maureen was tired for a week to ten days. That is probably a natural reaction to the trauma in the surgery and recovery. But now she is back in the groove of rehabilitation. Her therapists—physical, speech, and occupational—are doing their thing three times a week, and there is improvement in all areas.

The home therapy will end soon. Maureen will start on out-patient therapy at the Davies campus of California Pacific Medical Center on the 27th. The home therapists were very good, but so were the people at Davies, and I am sure that Maureen will enjoy being back with them. Those who have not seen Maureen for a while are all very surprised at her improvement. She still has a long way to go, but when you see her after having not seen her for a while, it's pretty heart-warming, She still has some difficulty in grasping how to say "that word" that is in her head, but she finds ways to overcome these difficulties, using other methods of communication to make up for the shortcomings. And there is constant improvement

Some friends have told me they were not sure if they should telephone Maureen, they were not sure that she could handle it. Well, she can. She talks to her Aunt Marge, who is famous in the annals of Pacific Telephone history, every day (family joke!). It occasionally takes a modicum of patience when she gets stuck on a word, but, overall, she does very well. In case you forgot, her number is 415-___-____.

Maureen has also expanded her social life. She was out three nights this week, with friends Monday and Wednesday and with family on Thursday. What was once a problem has become a slight inconvenience. Maureen can handle it well.

Thanks to all of you for your concern.

—Jack & Judy Twomey

But on December 22, 2000, I had a seizure again.

I was at home, sitting with MaryAnn and Chuck, when I started to feel weird. And then I had a seizure. I can't remember much about this one, but MaryAnn and Chuck did.

Epileptic seizure signs and symptoms:

The signs and symptoms of seizures vary depending on the type. Seizures may cause involuntary changes in body movement or function, sensation, awareness, or behavior. Seizures are often associated with a sudden and involuntary contraction of a group of muscles and loss of consciousness, a brief or long-term loss of memory, or a sensation of fear and total state of confusion. Seizures are typically classified as motor, sensory, autonomic, emotional or cognitive. After the active portion of a seizure, there is typically a period referred to as postictal before a normal level of consciousness returns . . .

Dr. Kitt tried a different medication for me this time, Lamictal. I didn't have an allergic reaction to this one. "Hopefully this will work," I thought.

Kevin (my brother), me (shoooooortest hair), and Judy and Dad.

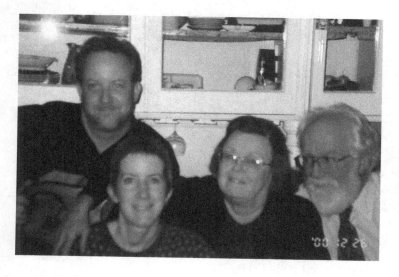

MaryAnn, some gray-haired woman (oh wait, the gray-haired woman is me), and Chuck:

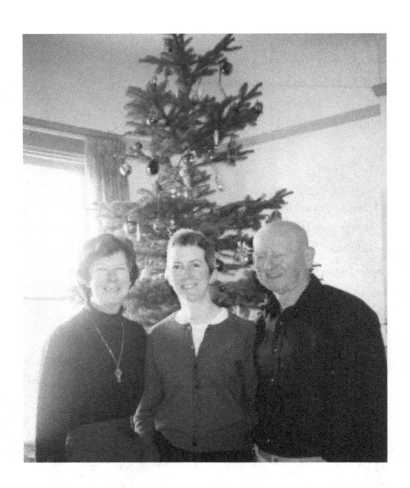

(In January, no more gray hair!
"Hey, I need some I.D.")
;)

(Chapter 19)

January 2001

Ad firms were laying people off in 2000 (the bursting of the dot-com bubble). So in January, GMO/Hill Holliday had to lay fifty people off.

I thought I still worked at GMO/Hill Holliday, however, even though I knew I was not getting a check from them anymore, and I now had COBRA.

> **COBRA:** A measure to give departing employees the option of temporarily continuing to purchase health insurance through their former employer.

Somehow, I thought I still worked there, and that when I was better, GMO/Hill Holiday would take me back.

More on that later . . .

❀   ❀   ❀

I wanted to do Avon's breast cancer
walk in July 2001 since I hadn't been
able to do it in 2000. But so far, I could
only walk maybe four blocks, and it
took me twenty minutes or so to do it.

Rrrrrrrr . . .

❀   ❀   ❀

In February 2001, I was finally able
to write a full sentence alone. (I can't
remember what I wrote, but it was
longer than "I sit.") It's amazing that it
took me so long, but I did it.

I was watching TV one day, and a
doctor on the show I was watching said,
"If you had a brain accident, stroke,
etc., for the first three to six months
afterward you will see improvement.
But after six months . . . sorry."

HAAAAA! It took seven months
before I could read one sentence
alone. But I stuck with it, and
eventually I was doing it.

So, Doctor—you're wrong! SNAP!

❀   ❀   ❀

March 22, 2001: My B-day
MaryAnn and Chuck had a party for
me—family and friends. I said thanks
to everyone for coming. At the party,
I said, "Two weeks from now or less, I
will be 100 percent better."

(Yes, I was kidding.)

I was supposed to finish with PT,
OP, and speech on March 31, 2001 or
so, but they extended my "stay." So I
continued at Davies.

Kevin, me (bad hair day, so I covered
my face), Mom, and David DiLullo (a
friend):

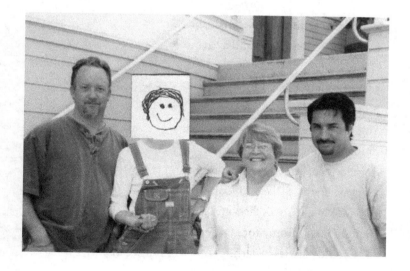

Mike, Joan, and Yogi at their
house (First time I took a picture since
my stroke—man, I take great pictures!
I should be a full time photographer
now!):

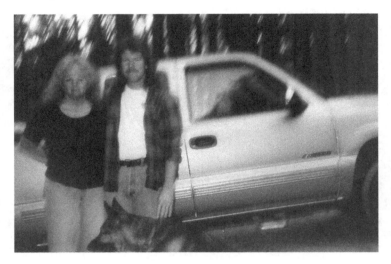

Kind of funny story: Mike and
Joan have a dog (Yogi) and a cat
(Plop). One time a day, when I was
sitting at their table, I took off my
brace and did some exercises, and
Yogi was so interested in what I was
doing. I thought, "I'm really not
doing much, but you're watching me
anyway, Yogi?" Mike and Joan were
also looking at Yogi's face, and they
thought it was funny too. Of course,
Plop could care less. Darn.

❀　❀　❀

I had two more seizures. The first
one was in February 2001. When
it happened, Dr. Kitt increased my
Lamictal dosage. The next was in
March, 2001, and Dr. Kitt increased
the dosage again.

I had *another* seizure in May
2001. I had forgotten to take my pills
the day before, and I hadn't taken the
pills yet that morning. I was sitting on
the chair in the shower and had just
turned the shower off when my right
arm began swaying really fast (kind of
like a rave dance from the '80s dance,
but NOT fun).

MaryAnn was just outside of
the bathroom, and we were the only
ones at home. I said, "Why is my arm
twitching . . . HELP." And then it was a
full-blown seizure.

MaryAnne came into the
bathroom and helped me. She kept
saying, "Lord God Almighty, help her."

Chuck came back and MaryAnn
yelled for him to come upstairs. The
seizure was over, but I was out of it.
(MaryAnn said later that the seizure
lasted for a minute or so.)

MaryAnn quickly put the towel

around me and got Chuck to carry me into the bedroom.

(I remember in September of 1999, I was walking through a park in Rome with two friends, and we decided to go to the Vatican. As we walked past an older couple sitting on a bench, the man began to have a seizure. The woman was yelling for help. One of my friends quickly helped them, but I was frozen. I was thinking, "Oh my gosh. I hope I never have a seizure, I couldn't deal with it.")

"I can't take it anymore!" I thought. "I shouldn't have done the surgery!" Yes, I knew I would still have to be wearing the helmet if I hadn't had the surgery, but wearing the helmet was better then having seizures. "Seizures are the worst!" I thought.

Dr. Kitt had increased my Lamictal three times already at this point, so after this seizure, he suggested I take the Lamictal plus Keppra.

"We'll see," I thought.

(Chapter 20)

One day, there was a phone call at the house. MaryAnn picked up; it was William J., who was still taking care of Salinger.

"How is Maureen doing?" he asked.

"Better every day," MaryAnn said.

They both thought that I was ready to take care of Salinger again. (Studies show that dogs and cats can heal, relax, and restore our health to us!) So the next day William and Robert came to our house (well, MaryAnn & Chuck's house), bringing Salinger! Thank you, thank you, and THANK YOU William and Robert for taking care of her!!

Robert, William, Salinger, and me:

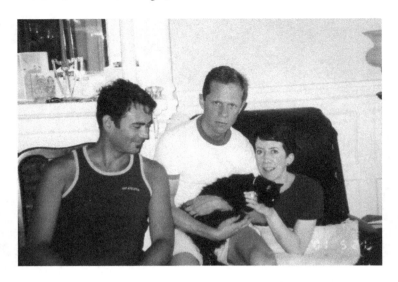

I was still seeing Deborah Van
Atta at Davies Campus, as well as a
reading instructor whose name I can't
remember. The reading instructor
gave me a book, *Little Women,* to
read in June (it was a really short
edition, but still, I finished the book—
whoohoo!).

It had been more than a year
since my stroke, and I still couldn't
walk without my right leg brace. So I
couldn't wear most of my shoes on my
right foot. I could have just kept every
pair of shoes that I had, but I gave

them to other friends and donated them instead.

Thankfully there are now some shoe stores where, if you have one shoe smaller and the other shoe bigger, you don't have to buy four pairs of shoes, you can just buy two.

Thanks, shoe people.

July 4, 2001, we were at a friend's party in Berkeley in the early afternoon. You could see the bay, so if we stayed until 9:30 p.m., we could see the fireworks.

Well, we were going home to San Francisco instead. I know there's fireworks in S.F. too (duh!), but you couldn't see them at Chuck and MaryAnn's house. So we went to Russian Hill. We arrived at 9:00 p.m. and got the perfect view. And thirty minutes later, the fireworks began . . . "Whoohoooooooooooo!" I thought. "This is soooooooooooooooooooo much better than last 4th of July!"

(CHAPTER 21)

Some more work I did with Deborah
Van Atta:

Dear Dad,   7/17/01
    Hello Dad! How are you?
I am great! It is sun___,
warm, and (nite). Well, I am
goes out. ___. See you soon!
                    Love,
                    Maureen

I meant to spell some of the words
wrong. . . . Just kidding.

In case you didn't realize what
I was saying there, here's the correct
words.

(sunny) (nice) (going) (duh)

(7/24-30/01)

Dear Mary Ann and Chuck,

Hi!

grateful
I am so ~~greatful~~ to
you!!!|||||

So tell me, how are
you? Well?

You nee—
(Vanitson)!!

So, go and (va———)!!|

Love,
Maureen

(need a vacation) (have a
vacation)

(Maureen . . . Oh wait! I got
THAT one right.)

8/2/01

Hey. Well I don't know ~~to~~
was to write — so, MMMM.
In time I will be 100%.
So (many) frien are so
dear to me I am so ~~much~~
grateful.
And in time I will help you!
Wooooo!

I think I wrote this one to YOU.
;-)

The following letter was only an
exercise, not a real job I wanted to get.
I wrote it in August 2001:

Dear Sir,

I would like to work for you. I have so much to __ . __

So I would like to get to (gether) we you.

I am at the phone (nu) 1-415- - .

I (ope) to here come you.

Sinel___
Maureen Twomey

(give) (together with) (number is)
(I hope to hear from) (Sincerely)

Good thing I didn't give this to a real employer. But why would I? I thought I still worked for GMO/Hill Holliday.

(Haaaaaa!)

By the way, at this point, whenever I wrote something, I had to speak out loud to hear the sounds of the words I was writing. For instance, I could spell these words correctly: how, you, great, warm, tell, write, friends, help, would, work, much, phone, here.

But if I wrote those words silently, without saying them out loud, I would spell almost every one wrong. Weird. "Well, in time I will not have to speak out loud when I write," I thought . . .

Around this time, I was at a party and was listening to a conversation two other people were having nearby.

One of them (I didn't know her) said, "That's nice she is doing better. I'm glad to hear that, but I'm not sure she will get much better."

?!?

(Side note: Yes, I'm mostly listening to another conversation, but yes, I can hear you talk too if you are not whispering!)

After we left, I said, "Was she talking about me?"

"Yes, Maureen."

"Does she think, 'It's been a year since the stroke, so she will mostly stay the same'?"

"Don't worry about her, Maureen. You are far better now than you were. Even now, I think you're more accomplished than she is."

A little later, in September 2001, I went to see Dr. Kitt.

"I don't know how far you will go," he told me, "because you have already gone beyond my expectations!"

HAAAA!!!

"I'm glad to hear that, but I'm not sure she will get much better."

Take that, lady! Snap!

I hadn't flown since the stroke. I had my first seizure in October 2000, and hadn't had another one since the last one in May 2001. Since I hadn't had a seizure for more than five months, Dr. Kitt felt I could fly again.

So Dr. Kitt wrote a letter for me:

Donald C. Kitt, M. D.

September 25, 2001

To Whom It May Concern:

Ms. Maureen Twomey is under my neurological supervision for a seizure disorder, for which she receives two medication named Lamictal and Keppra. She has a seizure disorder as a result of brain injury, for which she had major intracranial surgery in June of 2000. She has four titanium clips as a result of the surgery.

Ms. Twomey is safe to fly on an airline for a long period with good compliance with her medical regimen.

If you should have any further questions, please don't hesitate to contact me.

Sincerely yours,
Donald C. Kitt, M.D.

On Thursday, October 18, 2001, I was flying down to Los Angeles. When I got to the airport in SFO, someone had a wheelchair waiting for me (I could walk, but not fast). One of the airport people pushed me to my gate (thank you, airport person!).

I had Dr. Kitt's letter to take with

me every time I flew. Still, every time my metal clips set off an alarm, some lady would pat me down. Oh, what fun.

I was staying at Stephanie Barlow's house, so Stephanie, Steve, and Beth Callaghan picked me up at the airport. We were walking to the Cheese Factory later on and Steve was talking but I was distracted. "Who's walking so slow?!" I wondered. Then I realized it was ME. Haaaaaaa!

Friday I went back to TBWA\Chiat\Day (not TBWA/Chiat/Day) and got my old job back. (Kidding about the job.) It was so great to see everyone!

Later Stu Gibbs had a party at his house. I loved seeing everyone there. But maybe an hour and a half later, I suddenly thought, "I'm SOOOOOOOO tired! Can I go home now even though everyone is still here?"

Well, twenty minutes or so later, two people said good-bye to me. Some time after that, some other people said good-bye. Then two other people were going to go, so finally I whispered to Stephanie, "I'm soooooooo tired . . . can we leave?"

(Thanks, Stu and everyone else, for being so kind when I left my party earlier than the rest of you!)

Saturday, my friends Liz Pratt (Peanut) and Chris Gipson got married. It was a gorgeous wedding. After the ceremony, when we were at the party, I said to my friend Monika, "Can I steal this for when I get married?"

Someone else said, "Are you engaged?"

"No, I don't have a boyfriend yet, but that's not that important," I said, kidding.

When I got back to San Francisco, I forgot to mail this letter to Stephanie. Is it too late to send it now?

Oct. 22/01

Dear Stephanie,

Hey! Thank you for everything! 😊 I had so much fun. So who is going to get married next??

Well anyway, see you soon!

("So who is going to get married next?" Answer: Stu Gibbs and Suzanne Patmore Gibbs)

(Obviously, most of you reading this book right now got a different answer.)

(Chapter 22)

I was done for now at Davies Campus. But Sonya Richardson (PT) and Carolyn (OP) gave me plenty of exercises to do.

Deborah Van Atta gave me and Ellen Gilbert, M.S., this letter:

California Pacific Medical Center

Outpatient Department

SPEECH/LANGUAGE PROGRESS REPORT FOR THERAPY EXTENSION

PATIENT NAME: Maureen Twomey   DATE: 11/12/01

THERAPIST: Deborah Van Atta, MS CCC-SLP

SUMMARY OF PROGRESS: Pt continues to demonstrate success on meeting her goals, accepting each challenge with enthusiasm. She is now using strategies to provide and/

or record telephone numbers, including writing abbreviated messages. Ms. Twomey has expanded her ability to verbally communicate to include a group treatment class at John Adams community college. She recently completed her first trip to Los Angeles since her stroke. Reading and writing skills are also making steady gains. Ms. Twomey is beginning to read her second novel (designed for intermediate readers). She is writing short (3–5-word sentences) notes to friends with moderate assist for word retrieval. As word retrieval, reading, and writing continue to present the greatest challenge of therapy, pt has recently had a computer set up in her home for possible AAC purposes. She is starting to participate in exploring software options, such as word prediction software, as a possible aid to advance her writing skills.

PLAN OF TREATMENT:

1) With strategies learned in therapy pt will be able to reduce fillers, paraphasias, apraxic blocks, circumlocution, etc., 60% of the time using Melodic Intonation Therapy;

2) Pt able to read and demonstrate comprehension for intermediate level material with 70% accuracy, self monitoring for strategies;

3) Using adaptive software, pt will be able to type and send emails (5 sentences) with non dominant hand to familiar persons with 70% accuracy, mod cues for semantics/syntax;

4) Pt to perform Internet search on computer and to type basic information (name, address) required, with adaptive aids, mod cues, and 60% accuracy.

EXPECTED OUTCOME/GOALS:

Pt to maximize her rehabilitation potential for expression,

comprehension, reading, and writing in order to communicate within the unfamiliar community, using augmentation and assist as needed. Electronic aids will continue to be investigated and utilized as appropriate.

—Deborah Van Atta, MS

(Deborah, and later Ellen Gilbert, told me that maybe I would not reach 100 percent, but that there were many new programs that would help me with my reading and writing.)

I started with Ellen Gilbert, M.S. (she did speech, language, reading, writing, spelling, computer, etc.) on November 11, 2001. And thankfully, Ellen lived only a block away from Chuck and MaryAnn's house! Wow.

I went to see Ellen two times a week. At the beginning, she taught me the structure of the English alphabet using a chart that showed where all of our vowels and consonants come from.

I learned the sounds for the letters, and Ellen wrote each one on a chart that showed the consonants (single, blends, and digraphs) and the vowels (short, long, R and L controlled, and digraphs):

CONSONANTS

SINGLE	BLENDS	DIGRAPHS
s, p, n, d, m, k,	initial:	2 letters — 1 sound
c, j, t, v, f, r,	bl, cl, fl, gl, pl	ch, sh, th,
w, l, b, h, y,	br, cr, dr, tr, gr, fr,	wh, ph, ck,
z, x, g	sk, sl, sp, sw	tch, dge
	final:	
	ft, mp, nd, lk	qu

VOWELS

SINGLE LETTER SHORT/LONG		-r & -l Controlled	DIGRAPHS
ă = hat	a-e hate	ar (car) or (corn)	ai (rain) ay (play) ea (break)
e = pet	e-e Pete	er (her) ir (bird)	ee (feet) ea (eat)
i = bit	i-e bite	ur (burn)	ie (pie)
o = hop	o-e hope		oe (toe) ow (snow) oa (boat)
u = cut	u-e cute	all (ball) alk (walk)	ue (blue) oo (boot)
		al (bald)	ou (ouch) ow (how)
Short	Long		oi (oil) oy (boy)
			au (August) aw (saw)

ANGLO-SAXON LETTER-SOUND CORRESPONDENCES

M. HENRY 17

I also learned the spelling for different sounds, like /oi/ and /oy/. Then I wrote words with the sounds. Then I wrote a sentence with some of the words. Below you can see one of my exercises with those vowel digraphs and also the ending–*ture:*

oi (oil)	oy (toy)
- avoid	annoy
coin	coy
foil	employ
join	enjoy
noise	loyal
poison	oyster
sirloin	voyage
thyroid	
tinfoil	"She so coy ...
turmoil	I'll avoid her."
turqoise	100%

—ture (cher)

root word	suffix	new word
lec	-ture	lecture
pic	-ture	picture
cul	-ture	culture
struc	-ture	structure
rup	-ture	rupture
cap	-ture	capture
frac	-ture	fracture
fur-ni	-ture	furniture

"I was going to capture the
guy, but I ____ fractured my
leg."

❀ ❀ ❀

From: Jack and Maureen Twomey
Sent: 11/11/2001

Hi,
This is Maureen's Dad (Jack Twomey).

. . . Maureen is progressing in her therapy. She wants to use
e-mail to keep in contact with all of her friends. However,
her capabilities in writing are limited at the present time.
She can totally understand what is written to her, but it is
difficult for her to write to you. The whole process of writing
consists in thinking about what you want to say, then form-
ing that thought into language, then remembering how to
spell all the words you have chosen, then typing them on
the keyboard. Maureen has no trouble with the thinking
part, but she has to re-learn most of the rest of it. It is com-
ing along, but it is a lot to re-learn. But she will work hard
at it and it will come. In fact, Maureen is now sitting at the
keyboard, and has taken control of this letter . . .
    HEY!!! IS MAUREEN TWOOOOOOOOOOOMEY!!!
    :)
    I am sooooooo grateful to everyone—thank you.
    So sent me a letter!

Love,
Maureen

. . . My first e-mail since the
stroke, and I misspelled two words:
"It's" and
    "send."

Damn.

❀   ❀   ❀

I got my first workbook: *Explode The Code* by Nancy Hall and Rena Price.

Lesson 1 was c followed by *e, i, or y.*

Join the syllables to make a word that fits each meaning. Use your dictionary to help you.

1.	cir cle cus	An animal show __circus__ A round, closed line __circle__
2.	test con cert	A race or test of skill __contest__ Musical entertainment __concert__
3.	ny cil pen	A one cent coin __penny__ Something to write or draw with __pencil__
4.	sauce apple cider	Stewed apples __apple sauce__ A drink made from apples __apple cider__ (two words)
5.	force ful peace	Quiet and still __peaceful__ Full of power __forceful__
6.	cess place re	To put back __replace__ A playtime between classes __recess__
7.	feat cide de	To make up your mind __decide__ To beat; to destroy __defeat__

Pick the best word to finish each sentence.

peaceful	~~cider~~	dancing
~~juicy~~	~~center~~	~~circle~~
~~pencil~~	~~circus~~	~~decide~~

1. When you do your homework, you need paper and a
   pencil.

2. It is exciting to go to the _circul_ to see the lions and trapeze acts.

3. _Cider_ is a great drink made from pressed apples.

4. Can you draw a _circle_ with a triangle in the middle?

5. Someday you will _decide_ what kind of job you want when you grow up.

6. Peaches and tomatoes are very _juicy_.

7. The pitcher stands in the _center_ of the baseball diamond.

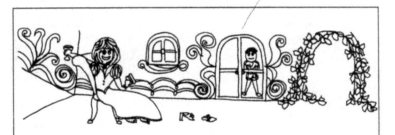

Ella Cinders had a chance to go to a fancy ball at the royal palace. She wore a lovely long, blue, lacy gown with a jewel necklace and a ruby red bracelet. Dressed up so splendidly, she looked like a real princess. The charming prince asked her twice to dance, but she would not. She decided she would rather relax, drink apple cider, and eat ice-cream sandwiches on the cool, breezy terrace. It was too hot to dance, her face felt warm, her glass slippers were too tight, and she hated the slow music. Why didn't they play rock and roll?

Answer the following questions. You may look back at the story.

1. Where did Ella Cinders go? *To the royal palace*

2. What was her gown made of? *blue lacy*

3. How many times did the prince ask her to dance? *twice*

4. What did she eat and drink? *ice-cream sandwiches and apple cider*

5. Why did her feet hurt? *because her feet were to tight*

6. What kind of music did Ella like? *rock and roll*

"TOO, not TO . . . duh, Maureen."

❀   ❀   ❀

I saw Chris Chandler and Wayne
at Davies Campus again, I think in
November of 2001.

I said, "I really thought by now I wouldn't have to wear my leg brace. On the other hand, I think my walking is faster now?"

They were more concerned about my knee . . . it was still locking back. They decided I needed a longer brace that would go above the knee.

"What!?" I said. I thought I was getting better, not worse.

"No, that's not the problem," Chris said. "Your knee is locking back, even with the Swedish Knee Cage. So if I don't fix the problem, the knee will get worse."

So Chris said he would make me a new brace—one that was higher but would mean I would never have to wear the knee support, so if I had long pants on, no one would be able to tell I had a brace on.

Alright. :-1

(Chapter 23)

In December 2001, Chuck and
MaryAnn had a party—a very fun
one. I went to bed late and woke up
at maybe 6 a.m., when I realized that
I hadn't taken my seizure pills (I was
supposed to take them every morning
and evening).

Aaaaaaah! I quickly went
downstairs and took my pills, but
I was still worried I was going to
have another seizure, so I woke up
MaryAnn (she was a nurse, after all).

MaryAnn didn't think I was
going to have a seizure, but she said
she'd call the doctor's answering
service (it was still early in the
morning, so Dr. Kitt was not going to
be in the office . . . duh).

Dr. Kitt called back and talked
to MaryAnn. "It has been more than

seven months since her last seizure," he said. "She only forgot to take her pill this once; tell Maureen not to worry."

SPOILER ALERT:
Never again have I had a seizure.
Yeah!

But hey, I have now mentioned Lamictal and Keppra several times in this book. Maybe they should pay me some royalties!

How about it, Lamictal and Keppra? Mmmmmm?

December 2001
Merry Christmas!

There is a line about it being lucky (or maybe it was unlucky) living in "interesting times." Well, we are definitely living in interesting times. It is difficult to begin to comprehend what happened in June 2000. It has changed all of our lives, our expectation of living a normal life, even if we go on doing most of what we were doing before. The background is different. There is now a firmer realization that the totally unexpected can happen at any time and at any place, and it might involve us or someone close to us.

Of course, the totally unexpected is what happened to Maureen. But she has survived, she is out of danger, and is progressing every day. She can now walk without the use of a cane. She still wears a brace on her right leg, but she has been testing her ability to walk without the brace. She has recovered feeling on her right side, especially the leg, but there are also signs of feeling in her right arm. Some of the feeling is painful, but that is part of the bargain. She can walk up and down stairs without the cane.

Her speech is progressing. She still has some difficulty remembering how to say "that correct word," but that difficulty is subsiding steadily week by week. Her speech has become much more facile. She is getting good speech therapy and is working hard at it.

She continues developing writing with her left hand. She has just recently gotten back on her computer. There is a lot to learn there. There are several processes involved in writing a letter on a computer, separate parts that we don't even think about, and she has to re-learn all of them. They were all left-side skills. But she has no difficulty with what we consider the basis function of the brain—thinking. And her memory is very good.

Best of all, she works really hard at her rehabilitation, going to her therapies and doing all of the homework involved. And she still has a positive attitude that is strong enough to face up to the difficulties that still exist. It may take another year, maybe more, but I am convinced that she is going to come all the way back. And I am certain that she believes the same.

All of us, Maureen included, greatly appreciate your concern for her, your prayers, and good wishes.

—Jack

❀ ❀ ❀

I sent this Christmas card to my
friends, family, doctors, nurses, and
therapists that year:

One year and a half ago (June 6th and 7th,
2000) I got sick – reallyyyyy sick. I almost died.

But, because of you, Doctors, Nurses and
Therapists – Emergency, In-patient and Out-
patient – Friends and Family – I lived.

I can't thank you enough.

Really – thank you.

Love,

Maureen Twomey

(It's not funny, but it is
appropriate.)

So I did a second card too:

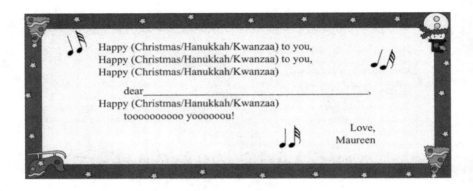

Happy (Christmas/Hanukkah/Kwanzaa) to you,
Happy (Christmas/Hanukkah/Kwanzaa) to you,
Happy (Christmas/Hanukkah/Kwanzaa)

dear_____,
Happy (Christmas/Hanukkah/Kwanzaa)
toooooooooo yooooooou!

Love,
Maureen

I know that the Christmas trees, snowman, and sleigh on this card are upside down; the images on the other cards were right side up, but I gave them all away to everyone else, so I only have this card now. Sorry.

Anyway, maybe it's not the best card, but *I* did it.

P.S.: You can write YOUR name up there on the card if you want to too!
;)

(Chapter 24)

GMO/Hill Holliday again . . .

Kathy Looney and I were at a coffee shop, and a friend came in who had worked for GMO before and now had a new job.

I said it sucked that I'd had a stroke in June 2000, but when I was better I'd go back to GMO/Hill Holliday.

"I don't have money from GMO/Hill Holliday because I'm not working yet," I told her, "but in time I'll get better, and I can return to work."

(?)

Later in 2002, I called a friend at work one day and said, "I'm trying to get back to work as soon as I can . . .

I'm making progress with reading and writing, but I'm not ready to come back yet. I'm so sorry!" I think I almost cried.

My friend didn't know what to say . . .

Courtney (she was the H.R. lady, very friendly) called me soon after and invited me to lunch. When we got to the restaurant, right away she said something like, "You still have COBRA, but you no longer work for GMO/Hill Holliday."

"Oh, duh, Maureen," I thought.

Later I called my dad. He had all my files (from GMO/Hill Holliday, Wells Fargo, etc.) because I still couldn't read or write that well.

I said, "I don't work for GMO/Hill Holliday anymore, it turns out."

He also thought I still had a job. Oh well. :-l

I was getting somewhat faster at walking; when I was walking down a street one day, I passed three other people who were also walking in that direction! Of course, I think they were seventy or eighty years old; when they were in their thirties, they were probably much faster than me.

In San Francisco, if you don't know this already, there are tons of hills. I lived in a flat area, but three blocks away there were tons of hills, and two blocks the other way there was a ton of traffic. So I got a stationary bike at home in March 2002:

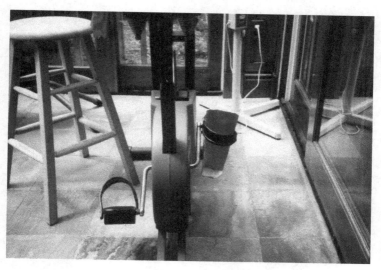

The OP made this foot thing for the right peddle, so my brace couldn't get stuck. "Man!" I thought. "I finally can bike fast again! Whoohooo!"

In September 2001, I had joined a stroke and brain injury group that met at John Adams campus on Fridays from 10-12 p.m. to talk about issues we were having. I was the second-youngest person in the group.

Some topics we discussed:
- Tips for Stress Management
- Know Your Triggers
- *When Music Heals* by Oliver Sacks

In spring 2002, Sharon, the group leader, said we should do a book about every person in the group. And so we did:

WHO WE ARE

SPRING SEMESTER 2002

We are in a San Francisco City College class for those who have had a stroke or other brain injury with language problems.

We are great!

We come from all walks of life. We are young, we are old, we come from all categories of race, religion and the world. We make up a very beautiful bouquet.

We come to class once a week to improve our communication skills.

We have learned that life goes on despite our infirmities. We as a group have vast knowledge. We can talk about everything and someone in the group knows about it.

We get great knowledge by sharing our experiences together and by becoming a personal group.

Our field trips are an added benefit.

We are all getting better because we are not alone. We want to better our condition. We encourage each other. We become stronger by the camaraderie we have with each other.

Come visit us and before you leave you will have learned something.

Written by the students enrolled in the course "Acquired Brain Injury Language Reintegration", a non-credit course offered in the Disabled Students Program Services Department, John Adams Campus, San Francisco City College. This course is taught by Speech Pathologists.

Here's what I wrote about myself
(someone else helped me write my
page, but I did write it!):

My name is Maureen Twomey. I was born in Santa Clara, California. I obtained a Bachelors of Art degree in Communications in 1990 from the University of California in Los Angeles. I worked for an advertising firm as a copywriter.

My family consists of my dad and stepmother Judy, my Mom and my brothers Mike and Kevin and my sister in law, Joan. I live with my Aunt Maryann and my Uncle Chuck.

I was working as a copywriter when I had a brain injury. I have had to learn basically everything over again; walking, speaking and reading.

In my free time I read, write, bike for thirty minutes per day, do arm and leg exercising and practice walking without a brace.

Well, one thing is that my sense of humor is still intact! I want to tell others who have had a brain injury or a stroke that family and friends are essential. It is hard work—REALLY hard work. But, I think everyone in my group is getting better. It's amazing!

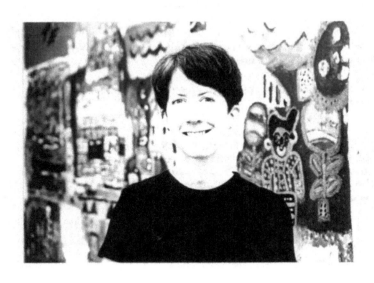

("... bike for thirty minutes per day"?? More like three times a week. But hey, sometimes I'm too busy ... so sue me.)

I said "brain injury" because at this point I thought what happened to me wasn't a stroke after all. In the hospital I'd thought it was a stroke, but then some people had told me, "It's similar to a stroke, but it's not a stroke."

Finally, Dr. Kitt told me, "Yes Maureen, it WAS a stroke."

I think when this book is finally published, some other important people still will insist that what happened to me was not a stroke. But if that's you, I hope you don't get too mad to finish this book! Please, continue to read.

;)

(CHAPTER 25)

The computer: I didn't want to take the "easy way out" when I first started to relearn how to read and write. After all, I now knew that you could hit a key (see right below how to do it . . . if you didn't know already), and the computer would read what I wrote back to me.

To turn on talk on a Mac computer, you click "System Preferences," then click "Speech," then "Text to Speech." Apple has twenty-three voices you can choose. Some of them are funny. (I chose "Vicki.") Once you select a voice, you check "Speak selected text when the key is pressed," then click "Change Key" and choose they key you want to use to activate text to speech. I chose F1.

How do you turn on the voice in Microsoft Windows? I don't know. Hmmmm . . . Oh, I called Kevin, and he said, "It's Control Panel, and then double-click Speech." (Thanks, Kevin.)

"Isn't it nice to have a computer that will talk to you?" the computer said to me.

I could just open a new document, write some stuff, and then "Vicki" would read it back to me. Of course, I was limited in word choices, so I couldn't write much. Hmmmmm.

Ellen Gilbert suggested that we start trying out some programs (like Don Johnston© Co:Writer) and see where those went.

So what is Co:Writer (and Write:OutLoud)?

"Co:Writer is a predictive word software program designed to assist people with writing difficulties. Those with physical access issues or difficulties with written expression may benefit from the use of this "writing coach." Co:Writer allows users to write complete sentences with very few key strokes. As you type a letter, Co:Writer produces a list of predicted words. As you continue to add letters to the word, Co:Writer refines the predicted word list . . ."

"Alright," I thought, "I'll try it."

With Co:Writer, you write sentences one at a time. As you begin to type a word, Co:Writer offers guesses as to what the word is, based on the letters you've typed and on other factors. If the word you want is in the list of guesses, you select the word and continue to the next word. If the word you want is not on the list, you continue typing until it is, or until you finish the word. When you finish your sentence, Co:Writer "sends" it to your word processing program, Write:OutLoud.

This is what using Co:Writer looks like:

I

1: Is
2: I
3: It
4: Isn't
5: In

It i

1: is
2: isn't
3: invites
4: in fact
5: imagines

It is to
1: today
2: to
3: tomorrow
4: told
5: too

It is too h
1: hard
2: happy
3: hot
4: huge
5: hungry

It is too hot to
1: to
2: today
3: tomorrow
4: too
5: tonight

It is too hot to g
1: go
2: get
3: going
4: give

It is too hot to go an
1: and
2: an
3: anymore
4: anyway
5: anywhere

It is too hot to go anywhere
>   **1: but**
>   **2: and**
>   **3: to**
>   **4: a**
>   **5: the**

. . . The program keeps giving me options, but I'm done with my sentence, so I hit the period, and Co:Writer immediately imports it into my Write:OutLoud document, which now says:

"It is too hot to go anywhere."

Whoohooooo!

(Wait, I'm in San Francisco . . . when DOES it get too hot, anyway?)

Some things I did with Co:Writer and Write:OutLoud:

-Wrote about San Francisco places to visit

-Practiced prepositions

**-Wrote about stroke stuff
etc.**

http://donjohnston.com/writing
http://donjohnston.com/writeoutloud

One day, a friend of mine said, "Your speech is coming back. And it will continue to come back as you speak more. But Maureen—before you had your stroke, you talked SOOOOO fast! Now that your speech is coming back, remember, don't speed up your words again!"

"Oh! Sorry . . . I will remember that now," I said.

❀ ❀ ❀

Chris Faber (a friend I met in my beginning improv class in February 2000) and I went to see a BATS Improv show on a Saturday in October of 2002.

Chris was in the Sunday night show now. I told him I thought I was ready to come back to the improv class—maybe not the intermediate class, but I could start over in the beginning class. But Chris thought I should take Laughing Stock first (an offshoot class). Jonathan Goldman, a guy I'd met in the intermediate improv class also did Laughing Stock:

"Through the Laughing Stock program, BATS Improv offers free improvisation classes to people living with HIV, AIDS, Hepatitis C, cancer, and other chronic, life-threatening illnesses. The classes focus on strengthening quality of life through humor, physical activity, group interaction, risk-taking, and imagination games. It is a safe and confidential environment for participants to learn the basics of improv. It's not stand-up comedy or drama therapy; it's an improvisational theatre workshop for folks with all levels of performing experience."

TESTIMONIALS: Here's what some past students have said about Laughing Stock classes:
- "A Blast! The coach was a real scream!"
- "I learned the art of being silly."
- "Would have liked this to have lasted three times longer."
- "Gained increased self-confidence."
- "Now I can embrace failure."
- "A creative way to celebrate taking risks."
- "Why did I wait so long?"
- "New neurons developed."

A guy named William was teaching the class. Everyone was so easygoing and nice there, and I thought I would do well. But on the spot I couldn't think of anything! I used to be good at coming up with something on the spot, but I couldn't do it anymore. I felt like I was in the episode of *The Brady Bunch* when

Cindy Brady went on a quiz show. She was really smart, but when the cameras turned on, she froze.

I don't know why, but I got more insecure in this class. Now I was kind of crying ("Maureen!" I thought. "Get yourself together!")

"I think I should go," I told William. "Maybe I'm so tired that I can't think of anything . . ."

"Stay," William said. "You can be my assistant." He smiled.

"Okay!" (Thanks, William!)

I tried another Laughing Stock class sometime later (in 2004, I think?) with a different teacher. This time the class had a music-type theme . . . And again, when I was on the spot, I mostly couldn't think of anything. D'oh!

"Don't worry," the teacher told me. "When someone does a song and needs some backup singers, maybe you can do that."

So nice!

(Chapter 26)

In May 2003, I was at Davies campus, to do some more physical therapy when I saw Patricia Brill (she was in the Stroke Survivors Starting Over group and had visited with me in August 2000).

I think Pat was visiting some more people who'd had strokes that day. I was interested in what she was doing, and asked her how I could get involved.

Pat was so happy to hear that I was interested in joining the group. She had to visit with some more people that day, so she gave me her card, and I gave her my phone number and address (I didn't have a card yet).

On May 24, 2003, Pat sent me this letter:

May 24, 2003

American Stroke Association℠

A Division of American
Heart Association

Western States Affiliate
120 Montgomery St., Suite. 1650
San Francisco, California 94104-4319
Tel 415 433 2273
Fax 415 228 8402
http://www.heartsource.org

Dear Maureen,

I am so pleased that you are interested in volunteering with Stroke Survivors Starting Over! Your willingness to help other stroke survivors, as well as your energy and enthusiasm will be a welcome addition to the group.

I am sorry that we didn't have much of an opportunity to talk at the last quarterly meeting. Perhaps when Susan returns from her road trip, the three of us can plan to have lunch.

The training class will be held on September 15th from 1:00 pm – 3:00 pm in the volunteer office at Davies. The office is located on the same level as the cafeteria, Level T5. Also, it is possible that we will expand the training class to two

SESSIONS, IN WHICH CASE IT WOULD BE HELD ON MONDAY, SEPTEMBER 22ND AS WELL.

IF YOU HAVE ANY QUESTIONS, PLEASE CALL ME (TEL ▓▓▓▓▓). I WILL BE OUT OF TOWN FROM JUNE 10TH TO JULY 7TH. I KNOW THAT THE TELEPHONE MIGHT BE TOO DIFFICULT, BUT YOU CAN ALWAYS HAVE YOUR AUNT CALL ME WITH ANY QUESTIONS YOU MIGHT HAVE.

I AM LOOKING FORWARD TO SEEING YOU IN SEPTEMBER, IF NOT BEFORE.

BEST TO YOU,

PATRICIA BRILL

I started working with the group
in September 2004.

Maureen Twomey

Stroke Survivors Starting Over
Peer Visitor Program

My card; it also has my phone number on it, but I don't want to give YOU my number, so I covered it up. Haaa.

I started going to St. Mary's Hospital once a month (there were about fifteen other Peer Visitors, so obviously I didn't do it every week). I started with Barbara Combs, the woman who started the group after having a stroke. Another woman was Louise Rodriquez (she hadn't had a stroke, but her husband had, so she also volunteered). We teamed up too.

Some stroke patients that we saw seemed like they'd only had a miner stroke: their speech was fine and they could walk, etc. Some other patients had dysarthria.

> **DYSARTHRIA:** difficult or unclear articulation of speech that is otherwise linguistically normal.

I have some dysarthria too, but when I finally get my words out of my mouth, people understand what I am saying.

We were visiting St. Mary's one

day and saw a man who'd had a stroke and he had severe dysarthria; I mostly couldn't understand him. A month later, I saw him again, and he was talking so much more clearly. It was amazing.

I got Franklin, a Language Master, speaking dictionary, thesaurus, and grammar guide, and started using it:

www.franklin.com

I use Franklin to help with my spelling. If I type "Mauren," for example, Franklin says, "Correcting . . ." and then it gives me ten similar words. If you don't know some of the words, you can listen to them by pressing "Say." Here is one list Franklin gave me:

murrain

(The first word it gives me is *murrain?* That means "plague"!)

Maureen

maroon

Marian

Marianne

(I was not thinking of this, but Hi, Marianne! (That's my cousin.)

Marion

manure

(Hey! No, I was NOT thinking of this word!)

manner

meaner

Mainer

Of course, the one I wanted was
"Maureen" (duh), but now you can
laugh at some other choices that I got.

Maybe I should change my
name now, so you won't laugh at me?
Hmmmm . . .

(CHAPTER 27)

September 2003

I was going to start attending the stroke group at John Adams again, but instead I started eye exercises with Dr. Iole Taddei, an optometry specialist.

I still had difficulty with my peripheral vision on the right side. Looking straight ahead, I could see fine on my left but couldn't see anything on my right, which meant I couldn't drive . . . yet.

Dr. Taddei gave me several eye exercises to do to strengthen my eyes:

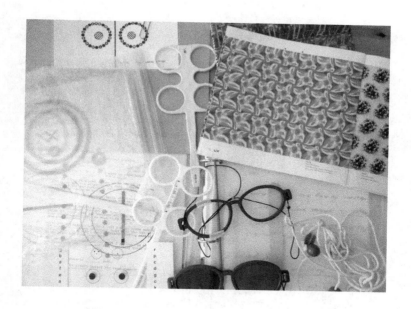

Meanwhile, the were more workbooks for me to complete, AND . . . my book!

"It took this stroke to get you to do the writing you always wanted to do," Ellen told me.

I started my book in November 2003 . . . Well, sort of. I thought I could explain what was wrong with me in maybe thirty pages or so. "Haaaa," I thought later . . .

I started out by using *Inspiration* to brainstorm. At first there were maybe five or six bubbles. I mostly just dictated to Ellen, and she typed what I'd said.

About the Inspiration views

Inspiration has two main views or environments: Diagram view and Outline view. As you work, both keep track of your ideas. Sometimes you will work exclusively in Diagram view to create a graphical organizer or a map showing how ideas or concepts interconnect. Other times you will work in Outline view where you might organize and write a report.

Here's what Diagram view looks like:

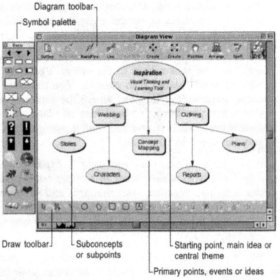

The Diagram view window

And here's what Outline view looks like:

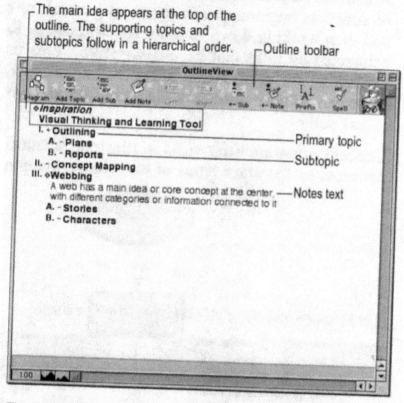

The main idea appears at the top of the outline. The supporting topics and subtopics follow in a hierarchical order.

Outline toolbar

Primary topic

Subtopic

Notes text

The Outline view window

(This is version 6.0, Grades 6 to Adult. Now it comes in version 9.0, http://www.inspiration.com/ Inspiration)

Gradually, I added more and more words. I didn't save the very first one, so here is the closest thing to the first one I can show you (I made it sometime in 2004):

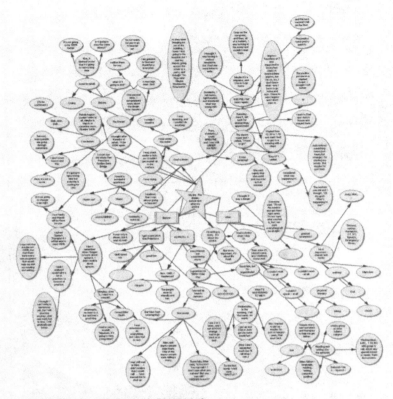

My life: The dream; before and after my stroke

I.   I'm writing a story. It's about my stroke.

    A.   But more important, it's about life itself.

    B.   I had a stroke when I was 33.

II.   I had a dream

What, you can't read it? Maybe
you just need new glasses. ;)

Anyway, I was really excited about
my book, but I still had a long way to
go . . . and plenty of other things I had
to do . . .

Christmas card, December 2003
(Hopefully this one is better):

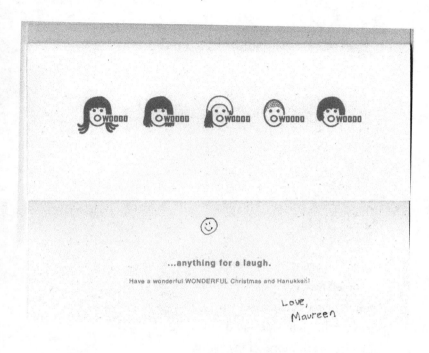

...anything for a laugh.

Have a wonderful WONDERFUL Christmas and Hanukkah!

Love,
Maureen

(Maureen Twomey, Copywriter,
Jenn Muranaka-Chaney, Art Director)

(Chapter 28)

February 2004

Back to the eye stuff: By February, Dr. Taddei felt that my eyes were much better. She gave me glasses with a prism on the right side—and now I could see much more on my right.

With the prism, you see two images at first. For example, if you were on my right and I turned toward you, I would see your image in the prism, seeming closer than you actually were. Then, farther away on my right, I would see the real you. After practicing (for a while), you see only one image. Once I was only seeing one image, Dr. Taddei felt I was ready to learn to drive again!

It had been four and half years since I had last driven—and now I had to learn how to do it all over again. I was so nervous! What if I hit someone!? AAAAAH!

On February 27, 2004, I started my training with Derrick Scott of APEX Driving School. Derrick's car had several adaptive devices; in my case, my right leg and right arm were limited and my left leg had to do the work—so the brake was on the right and the gas pedal was on the left. There was also a knob on the steering wheel so I could control the steering with one hand.

The car was also equipped with two sets of pedals (one on the left and one on the right side), so if I made a mistake Derrick could take over quickly (thank you, Derrick!).

"You can do it," Derrick said the first day. "Let's drive!"

The most important thing I had to learn first was: BRAKE IS ON MY RIGHT. GAS PEDAL IS ON MY LEFT. BRAKE IS ON MY RIGHT . . . etc.

The second thing I had to learn was to glance to the right more often—about every five seconds. If I didn't do that, I wouldn't see the right side at all, and that would NOT be good.

After those two primary things, I had to learn everything else (like keeping my eyes moving constantly).

Again, without my glasses, I couldn't see anything on my right side. The prisms in my glasses allowed me to see much further on the right side, and that, I think, is the only reason I was able to drive. If I didn't have the prisms, I would have run into someone after driving maybe half a block.

In time, Derrick felt that I could drive another car (one with no brakes on the right side).

I got my car April 8, 2004. Whooohooo!

(pictures of my gas and brake):

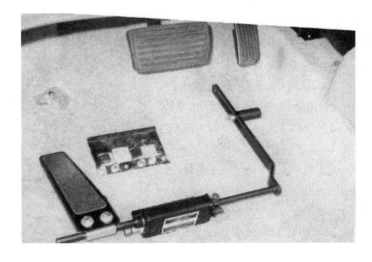

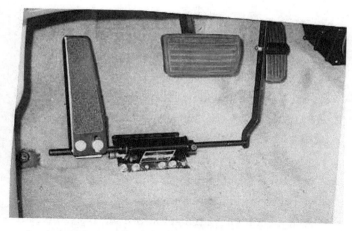

I got a parking placard, which meant that I could park in handicap spaces *AND* I didn't have to pay!! Of course, I would rather have not had a stroke, but it was nice that the DMV gave me the placard.

On May 4, 2004, Derrick felt I was ready to take the driving test. He wrote to the DMV:

Assessment Report 5/4/04

Driving/Subject: Twomey, Maureen

Vehicle: Left-foot accelerator and Steering knob mounted on the 10 o'clock position of the wheel. Subject is currently being trained in her own modified vehicle.

Traffic Conditions: Local residential and commercial traffic and freeways.

Observation Overview:

Ms. Twomey has demonstrated tremendous improvement over the course of her training. Ms. Twomey has a good overall skill level of the primary driving proficiencies: vehicle control, traffic rule adherence, and visual scanning.

Challenges in the training that must be taken in consideration if this driving privilege is disposed to DMV reexamination:

1. Due to the effect of her aphasia (which is primarily expressive and only mildly receptive), there may be some verbal communication miscues.
2. As it is common with many stroke survivors, there is the occasional directional confusion of left and right. This is a condition that may be exacerbated by fatigue, or when verbal instruction for a particular task lacks sufficient response time.

Current Training Objectives
- Visual scanning with specific attention to consistent use of mirrors and recognition-to-response to potential hazards within the traffic scene.
- Adapting scanning to compensate for vision loss to the right eye.
- Better tracking on non-stopping right turns.

Adaptive Equipment: Heavy-duty Spinner Knob (@ 10 o'clock, and left-foot accelerator.)

—Derrick Scott, Driving Evaluator

Apex Driving School
San Francisco, CA

I wanted to take the written test and driving test right away, but the DMV said I had to make an appointment.

"Oh," I said, "I have to wait for a week?"

"No," the woman said, "the earliest appointment available is on September 14."

WHAT??!!!!??

She explained some people have to go through more steps to get their license back; in my case, since I had issues with my peripheral vision, I needed someone with special training to test me. There was only one person that did this at the San Francisco DMV. So the first appointment available was not until September 14.

Alright.

So, for all of May, June, July, August, and the first half of September, I could have other friends ride with me, but never drive alone.

Finally, on September 14, I took the written test. I said to the woman at the DMV, "I had a stroke. I am significantly better now, but I still have trouble reading."

"There's an oral test you can take," she told me. Then she read me three questions. When she read the first question, she was talking kind of fast. I asked her to slow down.

She read it again. "Hmmmm," I thought. I needed time to look at all the answers, and so I had to read and select the answers myself. Many times, I would know one word, but not another word. In the end, I failed the test (D'oh!!!). But the woman was very nice and told me that I could take it again.

A week later, I passed the test. "Whoohooo!" I thought. I was sure I could take the driving test right after.

Not so. The woman said the earliest appointment available for the driving test was November 22. "AAAAAAAAH!" I thought.

Well, on November 22, 2004, I FINALLY passed the driving test (the first time I took it!). Thank you, Dr. Taddei and Derrick Scott!

"So, Maureen, are you driving every day now?" you ask.

Haaaa! No, I don't drive every day in San Francisco. I'm not very comfortable with busy intersections or busy streets still. I am more comfortable when someone else is in the car . . . then *they* can drive. (Just kidding . . . kind of.)

(Chapter 29)

May 11, 2005

I moved into my own apartment!

When you go on the roof on July 4th, you can watch two fireworks shows: one over the Golden Gate Bridge area, and one over the Bay Bridge area! (Well, I'm in San Francisco, so sometimes it's really foggy . . .

"Hey! I hear fireworks going off, but where are they?"

"'You see the clouds?'"

"Yes."

"The fireworks are up above the clouds.")

Anyway, back to my apartment. Some people thought, "How can you manage alone?" (with cooking, etc.)

I told them there's "Functional Solutions": Through them, I got some assistive dining products that I can use with one hand. For example:

- a Zim Jar Opener
- Good Grips knives
- a Good Grips cheese slicer

etc.

For bathroom safety, I had two grab bars installed to help me get in and out of the tub, as well as a shower chair.

I got my arm brace and my cane at the same place, too. Check it out if you want: www.BeAbleToDo.com.

Of course, some things are more difficult and/or too heavy for me to lift, and Functional Solutions doesn't come with everything (WHAT?!!). For those things, when someone comes over to my place, I say, "Will you help me with _____?"

(Thank you Kevin Twomey, Dad, Chuck LaMere, Matt, Patti(y) Caselli, and Jonathan Goldman, etc., as well as my friends in my building!)

❋ ❋ ❋

When I first started to work with Ellen Gilbert, I went to see her two times a week. After all, she was only a block away. But now I decided that it would be much better if I did more homework at home and not have to drive or take a bus two times a week to see Ellen. (Thank you for everything, Ellen!)

I still use "Vicki" on my MacBook, but I don't use Co:Writer or Inspiration anymore. Co:Writer is really good at helping with word choices and spelling, but I wanted to be better at doing it myself. So I just use Franklin, the Language Master, speaking dictionary, thesaurus, and grammar guide, now. And, of course, if I highlight words and press a certain key, "Vicki" will read what I wrote. If I spell something wrong I can hear the mistake and retype the word.

When I am online, and I see something I want to read but it's a somewhat longer article, I can highlight it and have "Vicki" read it to me instead of reading it myself. Maybe I should be practicing reading longer articles more on my own, but I'm doing several other things too, so this helps me.

(P.S.: If you e-mail something to me, don't worry about my sight problems: I mostly use "Vicki" for

reading e-mails, so she will tell me
what you said.) ;)

I was at a friend's house one day, and
a guy there was asking me about my
stroke: "But in time you'll be 100
percent again?" he asked.

"Well, I don't know if I will be 100
percent," I said, "but I'm getting better
all the time, so that's great."

But now he couldn't think of
anything to say.

"Hmmmm," I thought, "maybe
'He's just not that into you.' Oh well."

February 14, 2006
No one gave me roses or a gift for
Valentine's day; instead, some woman
hit my car . . . Oh, what fun!

I was in the second lane from
the right, and I was stopped because
the light was red. The right lane was
empty, and then there were cars
further parked on the side of the street
in the shopping area.

The light turned green, and I
began to go again. A woman was

going in reverse out of one of the parking spots and she didn't look behind her before pulling out—she just went for it, into the right lane and then into the left lane, where I was driving. I felt the bump and pulled over and parked.

We both got out of our cars, and when the woman saw that I had a brace on my right leg, she said, "HEY!! YOU SHOULDN'T DRIVE!!"

I calmly said, "I have a Adaptive Driving Aid for my handicapped car. I have the paperwork right here."

She was quiet now. "Haaa," I thought. I could tell she was at fault.

We checked both of our cars, and we saw no damage to either one.

"Alright," she said. Then she quickly left.

She was the one who was at fault, but now I was nervous, so I called Chuck and MaryAnn (I had just been at their house).

"Some lady bumped my car," I told them.

They could tell I was upset, so Chuck came and drove me home. (Thanks, Chuck!)

(Chapter 30)

September 15, 2006

(e-mail to my friends and family)

> I'm walk(ing) (not run(ning)) for the Heart and Stroke group, American Heart Association.
>
> Now, I probably will finish in last place, but I don't care. It is a great cause.
>
> Go to:
>
> https://www.kintera.org/faf/donorReg/donorPledge.asp?ievent=149304&lis=1&kntae149304=FD4F2C3E6E2B49D58B36BFB4CED86E32&supId=141003744
>
> :)
>
> —Maureen

What? "The Event that you are
trying to reach has been disabled"?
Well, here is what I wrote:
   "I am helping the American Heart
Association fight the nation's causes

of death by participating in the Heart Walk. Step out against heart disease and stroke by supporting my efforts. Please make a donation so I can reach my walker dollar goal.

. . . (Or MORE!)

Thank you for your support!"

(Thank goodness there were no hills there.)

The Heart Walk started at noon at The Embarcadero Plaza/Ferry Building and the finish line was at Pier 39 (I thought).

Jonathan Goldman and I started walking five minutes early to get a head start. When we got to Pier 39, I turned around and saw that there were TONS of people behind us. We'd finished, and I hadn't finished last! Whoohoooo!

Some volunteers for the Heart Walk were there, and they were saying, "You're halfway there!!"

"WHAT!?" I said to Jonathan. "I thought we were done now!"

"If you're tired, we can take a taxi back to the event instead," Jonathan said. "What do you think?"

"No, we can just walk back," I said. So we did.

I sent an e-mail when I got home:

Whoohoo! I finished the Heart Walk AND I didn't finish in last place!

Jonathan Goldman (my friend) finished last! — (well... kind of) (thaaaaaaank you Jonathan!)

(for letting me finish SECOND to last)

;)

And thank you to EVERYONE!

Love,
Maureen

Me and Jonathan at the Heart Walk:

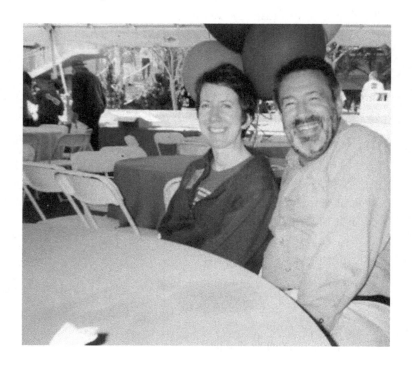

I did the Heart Walk again on September 18, 2009. But I started at 11:00 a.m. or so this time, and finished at 12:00 p.m., right as everyone else was just starting to walk—whoooohoooooooo!

"Next year and forever after, I will start earlier," I told myself.

:-D

I didn't work on my book much at all for a while—but in June 2007, I e-mailed some friends about my stroke, asking them, "When did you find out that I'd had my stroke?"

Heather Smith Siemons e-mailed me this:

> I think I found out the same day you went to the hospital. At the time, Andrew was married to my friend Fiona and he called me to let me know what was going on since he was working in the same office as you. After that day, Stephanie Barlow was really good about keeping me posted on how you were doing.
>
> How are things coming with the book? Hope you're enjoying putting it together—that's so much work!

Jenn Muranaka-Chaney e-mailed me this:

hey maureen!

whats happening!? ok, what i can remember . . .

david butler just got notice at work of what had happened
to you and had told me while we were sitting in our office. i
remember him giving what info he had and it seeming that
you not making it thru this stroke could be very likely. i was
in shock and to say i was upset was to say the least. i called
riki and she came over to our office and if i can remem-
ber correctly jill savage had happened to come by and saw
the tears and sat down too. we were all in shock, upset, had
questions, were confused.......it was painful since we were
not in san francisco and had to wait to hear of any further
news about your state of health.

it was the longest day ever.

i believe it was the next day or so your father sent an
email to everyone and to people at chiat on what had hap-
pened and what your state of health was. i remember read-
ing it and thinking "what does this mean!? . . . i don't know
what this means!". i think i was hoping for it end with "mau-
reen will eventually be fine." but it didn't. it was devastat-
ing...and we couldn't do anything at all to help, all we could
do was wait.

this is probably weird for you to read now, so many
years later and doing so well now! huh?

—l, jenn

Stu Gibbs e-mailed me back:

Maureen -

I don't really remember how I found out you'd had the stroke, which is strange. I do remember that you'd been in town just a few days before and that we'd all gathered at Stephanie Barlow's house to play games. As I recall, almost everyone there had been on "Win Ben Stein's Money." And then we must have watched the first "Survivor," because I actually associate that with the beginning of your stroke.

I was dating Jill at that time. I know that, when we found out about you, we were really just stunned. We had just seen you and you'd been completely fine—and now, there was this possibility that you might never be able to talk or walk again. We just kept wondering how that could happen to somebody. The word that comes to mind is "devastated." All of us: Me, Jill, Heather, Adam, Chris, Laura . . . We were devastated.

Your family must have been keeping us in the loop via email. I recall reading about how the stroke had occured—the biological aspects of it as well as the actually hows and whys of where you had been when it occurred.

I know Jill & I came up to SF maybe two weeks after the stroke and came to see you in the hospital. I don't think we were prepared to think that you really wouldn't be able to communicate with us. You could only really smile, nod and give a thumbs-up, so we had to sort of guess what you might like to talk about and hope we weren't boring you to tears. I know we told you about "Survivor." When we left, we were really hoping that you were going to get better.

And I remember that Mike Matthews thought it would be a good idea to get your improv friends to come perform for you. (Perhaps other people thought that, but I remember

Mike trying to make something happen.) And the story ultimately filtered back that you had spoken during that, telling your Mom to back off or shut up or something. Whatever it was, it was a great story, because it filled us with hope and made us think that you were going to fight back and become the Maureen we knew again.

I hope this helps.

—Stu

I remember Stu and Jill gave me
a fish . . . some other guy got the same
fish. Check it out:

http://youtube.com/watch?v=znd0tIKjsPU

Gail Curtis e-mailed me this:

Maureeena!

Are you writing a book? How exciting.

I do remember when I heard about your stroke. It was one week after the stroke happened—I was planning to come to San Francisco to visit you the following week. I don't remember who it was that called—or emailed. I was in shock and so scared for you.

So . . . I came to San Francisco and visited you at the hospital room instead! You were real sleepy when I saw you, with your little head all bandaged up. With all you had gone through, you still had your sense of humor intact—we were having a little laugh at a singing fish someone gave you.

Elaine B. Legere e-mailed me this:

Well, I can't remember the exact day, but I think it was when your dad sent out the email so it was at least a few days after your stroke—I think you were already stable, but obviously still in pretty bad shape. Fran and I were working at Palm in Santa Clara at the time, and she came over to my cubicle and told me. I think Dave had heard from someone, and I think he called your dad (?) and got on the email list so we could get updates about your health. I just remember how sad I was that you were going through such a terrible ordeal.

I remember during that time period, I was just sending out invitations to my wedding (which was August 12) and I didn't know if I should send you an invitation—I wanted you to know that I really, really wanted you to be there, but I also knew you were still going to be in the hospital, and I didn't want you to a) feel bad that you couldn't come, or b) worry about RSVPing or sending a gift. In the end, I think I sent the invitation with a note telling you that I wished you could be there, but you needed to take care of yourself first. That was a big memory for me, since planning my wedding was such a big project for me at the time.

Anyway, I hope that helps . . .

—Elaine

Many other people e-mailed back about when they'd heard I had a stroke as well (thank you all!).

"Okay," I thought, "now I will only concentrate on my book. So I think in six months from now, I'll be done!"

(HAAAAAAAAAAAAAAAAA!)

I went back to Davies campus for more arm and leg exercises:

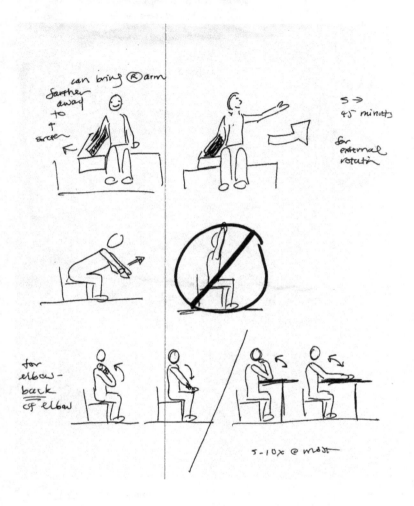

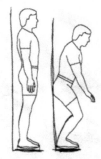

AROM knee squat bil w/cushion disk.

· Step up with both feet ~~onto cushion disk~~ on floor.
· Use wall or chair to obtain balance: Back to wall.
· Release wall or chair and bend knees into a squat, looking
straight ahead.
· Stand up and repeat.

Perform 2 sets of 10 Repetitions, once a day.

~~Use Wheel.~~
Rest 1 Minute between sets.
Perform 1 repetition every 4 Seconds.

Keep knees lined over toes

Sidelying knee lifts

* Lie on your left side, legs on top of
  each other

* lift your right knee away from the left,
  keep your feet touching   2 sets of 10

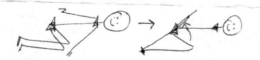

Issued By: Sonya Richardson, DPT   Signature: [signature]
These exercises are to be used only under the direction of a licensed, qualified professional.
CPMC   Except as to user supplied materials, Copyright 1995-2007 BioEx Systems, Inc.

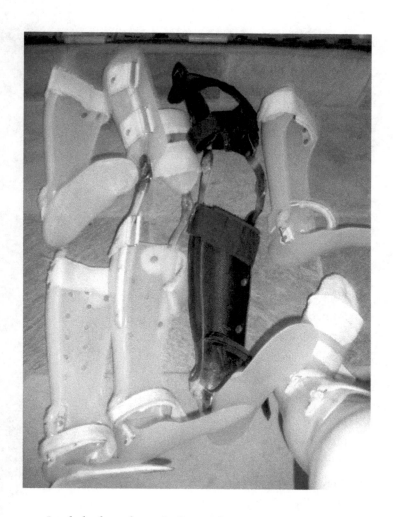

I only had one brace in September
2000. Now I have 6 . . .

I love San Francisco, but it has tons
of traffic (well, in L.A. there's MUCH
more traffic, but we still have a lot

here). So when I drive alone, I try to go on streets that have only one lane.

In July 2007, I was going to park in the St. Dominic's parking lot and was only driving five miles an hour when I scraped another car with mine . . . D'OH!!!!!!!!!!!!!!!

Thankfully, the other person was not in the car!! A friend of Chuck's saw the accident and ran over to me. "Are you okay?" he asked.

"I'm okay," I said, but I was thinking, "MAN, I'm so dumb!"

Someone else came over and he knew the person whose car I'd hit; he said he would go inside to get her.

The lady came outside, and I said, "I'm so sorry!"

Luckily, she was very nice. We got our insurance cards out, and when I called my insurance company they said they would take care of her car.

"I need to call Derrick Scott and tell him I need some more lessons," I thought.

❀   ❀   ❀

Two weeks later, I went down to L.A. to see Stephanie (Barlow) and Mark Kimura get married. ☺

That Sunday, I was at the airport,
waiting to go back to S.F. We finally
began to board the plane, but a lady
in front of me was attempting to fit a
huge bag, so I had to wait. It was kind
of funny watching her try to make
the bag fit. Anyway, another guy was
seated nearby, and he was looking at
me. "Hey that's Sean Penn," I realized.

Maybe he thought I was a famous
actress (haaaa). I had shorts on, so
everyone could see my brace on my
leg; maybe he was just thinking "What
happened to you?" Anyway, the lady
finally got the bag to fit, and she sat
down, so I was able to sit down. (Sorry
. . . not next to Mr. Penn . . . darn.)

(Chapter 31)

Now I go to Davies Campus to volunteer.

Every so often, the Peer Volunteer group meets. At one meeting, they gave us some magnets to keep and to give to other stroke survivors and their families:

Recognize stroke symptoms "FAST"

F FACE:	■ Uneven smile ■ Facial droop/numbness ■ Vision disturbance	**TIME SAVED = BRAIN SAVED** Fast medical and surgical stroke intervention can save your life and reduce disability.
A ARM & LEG:	■ Weakness ■ Numbness ■ Difficulty walking	**Call 911 immediately for emergency treatment**
S SPEECH:	■ Slurred ■ Inappropriate words ■ Mute	California Pacific Medical Center A Sutter Health Affiliate
T TIME:	■ Time is critical ■ **Call 911**	**www.cpmc.org/stroke**

It is so wonderful to have this on hand!

(Of course, I had every sign that I was having a stroke, so my friends called 911, I went to the hospital, and I got a CAT scan of my brain; but they saw nothing, because it was an artery in my neck. But again, more often it's the head.)

Google or Bing "FAST" stroke magnets to get some for yourself!

More homework . . .

Latin Roots:

leg (law, bind)

legal   legacy

illegal

legislate   legislation

legitimate   legislature

illegitimate

When he goes, the legacy that
you will get is his stuff animals! (?)

→ If you claim that President
Obama is illegal alien, you are
insane.

;-)

❀ ❀ ❀

I was looking at my Facebook and saw that some friends had done "25 Random Facts" about themselves, and now they wanted to know what MY list was.

At first I couldn't come up with twenty-five things, so I messaged them back, and said, "I can't think of 25 things! When I get done with my book, then I'll do them."

I went back to work on my book . . . "But how do I finish the third section?" I thought. After all, I had barely outlined the third part. D'oh!

"Maybe I should go do something else for while, and later, I'll come back to my book," I thought. "Yes!" So I went back to think of 25 things (VERY important stuff . . . not). Here's my list:

25 Random Facts About Maureen:

1) First book I wrote: *Sally The Snow Girl* (second grade)

2) The first kiss I got: He had braces in his mouth (I had them too). BUT he also had Oreo cookies in his mouth. Not good.

3) No really—the kiss was awful.

4) I was a Communication major at UCLA. I had good grades, but not honors. Lisa Puccini Brown (also Communication) went to a party (we were all wearing robes for graduation). Almost everyone else had special robes on. Lisa and I realized that we were the dumbest ones in Communication.

(Just kidding Lisa!)

5) I watched the *Real World* on MTV, Season 1. (1993 or 1994 I think). I loved it, so I mailed my form for the next one (in L.A.) to MTV. I had to write and tape (thank you Steve Callaghan) why I should be in it. Sadly, I didn't make it. Oh well.

6) I'm good friends with U2 . . . Then I woke up, and it was only a dream—I don't know them. :-(

7) Does someone know U2? If so, please let me know. :-)

8) My hair: I did have it longer, but the hair lady said, "You don't have the face for long hair." So I finally gave in, and now I have the same hair again.

9) June 5, 2000: Had a great time seeing a concert, Elliott Smith.

10) June 6/7, 2000: I had a stroke. Couldn't walk at all; couldn't speak at all; couldn't read or write at all . . . AAAAAAAAAAAAAAAAAAAAAAAAAH!

11) Hospital: Good people; bad food.

12) First words I said: Someone was telling a joke, but someone else was butting in. So I said, "BUTT OUT!"

13) Writing: The first word I wrote was "rav" (ravioli).

14) June 7, 2000, I could not walk at all, so I was in a wheelchair. I finally walked . . . alone . . . September 3, 2000. :-D

15) I still have a brace on my right leg, so I couldn't wear my shoes (the brace can't fit in my shoes). I gave the shoes to other friends and also donated them.

16) Maybe someday I will not have to wear the brace. So I'll call the people who have my shoes and say "I WANT THE SHOES BACK!!"
   ;-)

17) If I don't turn my head right, it is NOT because I don't like you; but now I cannot see on the right. BUT . . .

18) Now I have special glasses with prisms (right eye). So I can see much more . . . so now I have my license back! Beep Beep!

19) When driving, I use my left leg. So the brake is on the right, and the gas is on the left.

20) I liked wine and beer, but now I don't have the taste for it. So I have ice cream instead.

21) My family are all good or great cooks; I'm the only one who is not as good.

22) Please hold, your call is important .... Please hold, your call is important .... Please hold, your call is important .... Please hold, your call is important ....

23) Yeah for President Barack Obama!!!!!!

(John McCain and Mitt Romney are good people too though)

24) Hopefully I will finish my book soon . . .

25) Yeah, I'm done. (Not done with my book, only the list.)

Some friends posted comments:

Kassie Kehl Lewis:
#4 Hello! You graduated from UCLA—you are smart!!
#10 - #12 Wow
#18 - #19 again wow!
#25 - I am proud of you and I know so much more about you!

Duffy Smith:
I want to read your book. I want to read your book while eating ice cream. And even if you didn't have a special robe, you're one of the funniest people I know. (And I know funny!)

John Avery:

Nice Maureen. I love your list. And your courage.

Pam Edward:

I know U2 . . . oh that may have been in my dream too . . .

Greg Collins:

A near-minor correction on #12: I dunno if you remember or not, but when Greg Clancey and I came to see you in the hospital, in response to what was on TV, you couldn't say my name, but you almost said "Wimbledon." Congrats on having the stones to be around to type your 25, mama.

Rondi Walsh:

I had a huge treat today . . . coffee with Kassie. It was the first time we have seen each other since graduation. She clued me in to check out your 25. It has answered so many questions for me. Thanks so much for explaining so much of what I have missed in 25 lines or less. I am so impressed with your success. I am sure that it has taken a tremendous amount of work to get where you are. Ok, now you can keep entertaining me with your great sense of humor. Maybe you can fly down here and record an outgoing answering machine message for us?

Jim Mills:

Wonderful, your personality shines through here!

Maureen Twomey:

(Again, yea for "Speaking"/"Voice"
to say what I just said back to me.
So I can correct everything that I
spelled wrong.)

"Okay," I thought, "back to work..."

❀   ❀   ❀

More homework . . .

(Greek Roots)
    biblio (book)

    bibliography

    bibliophile

    bibliographer

AutoBibliography: AutoBiography
When I'm done with this
book, I will also write
★ that I've done:
   "Sally the Snow Girl" by
              Maureen Twomey, 1975
He is a bibliophile
★ guy. He doesn't read them,
   just collects them. Weird.

"He is a bibliophile guy . . ."
I TOO am a bibliophile, but I
really read (AND write) the books:

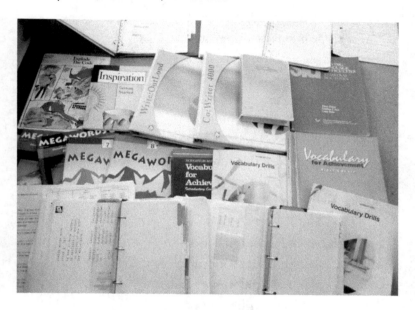

So there.

Some time later, when I was at Ellen
Gilbert's office, reading about what
happened to me again (Dad gave
me the letters that he had e-mailed
everyone else in 2000), I saw that
Dad had written in one e-mail that
one doctor said, "The damage is
permanent and irreversible."

"Permanent and irreversible!?" I

said. "I thought I'm much better now at reading and writing. So which is it?"

Ellen said, "He means that the damage to your brain is permanent, and that the brain itself is not going to reverse the problem on its own without surgery and therapy. There is always some spontaneous recovery after a stroke, but the doctor had only seen you at the beginning. That is how you looked at that time. He had no idea how much recovery you would have."

Hmmmm . . .

Well, because of the location of my stroke in my brain (left), the right side takes over. The right brain is much better at reading and writing now. But writing silently? That's the left brain. The right side needs to hear the auditory feedback for me to be able to put down what I want to say in writing. So basically, when I write I mostly have to speak the words out loud (still!).

I'm better at writing silently now though. Really.

Of course, if I write silently (I'll do it right now in this secetence), you can see I misspell a word—I can tell "secetence" is wrong, but I can't corrects it.

(I'm writing out loud now.) Wow
. . . I just listened again to what I
wrote. I only misspelled one word,
"sentence," but I should have said
"misspelled" not "misspell," and
"correct" not "corrects."

Oh well.

(Chapter 32)

Okay, I think I'm ALMOST done with this book now. When my book is done, maybe some people will want me to read parts of it out loud, and I will have to say, "Someone else can read it out loud." I can do it, but it would be slower. Yes, I really did write this book, but I'm not as fluent with reading and writing as many of you are . . . yet.

Maybe I will ask my friend Jenn Poulakidas to read my book out loud. She always laughs at my jokes; even if everyone else does not get my sense of humor, Jenn does. ;)

Of course, maybe 2 percent, I still think it's all a really strange dream . . . and I will wake up soon. I'm in my old apartment, I'm still thirty-three, and it's the morning of June 6, 2000. I haven't had a stroke, and nothing else is wrong with me (including my eyes, so that's why I can see all the way across the page).

But I have finally found a story to write a book about; it's not nonfiction, because I didn't have a stroke, so obviously it's fiction. It's a story of how I went to PMC for six weeks, then Davies Campus for eight weeks, then Aunt MaryAnn and Uncle Chuck's house for a few years, and then finally to my new apartment in May 2005.

When I'm finished with work today (June 6, 2000), I will work on my book—and I will finish it very quickly, because I'm 100 percent fine with my reading and writing!

I'm still walking the three-day walk for Avon this July, so I'll take a break from writing to go on a jog/run (after all, I don't have a brace on my leg, so I'm much faster and I can run as much as I want).

Oh! And I dreamed that something called "Facebook" will start up on February 4, 2004 . . . SO, if it's really June 6, 2000, *I* thought of it first! So . . .

(Well, if this is not a dream, I don't get any money from Facebook. Darn.)

Back to reality . . .

Checklist:

← ~~June 5, 2000 and Before:~~

~~Read:~~ ☑ ~~Yes~~

~~Write:~~ ☑ ~~Yes~~

~~Speak:~~ ☑ ~~Yes~~

~~Walk:~~ ☑ ~~Yes~~

~~Run:~~ ☑ ~~Yes~~

~~Drive:~~ ☑ ~~Yes~~

~~Good sense of humor:~~ ☑ ~~Yes (?)~~

~~Afdre~~ → Jd?! 6~@ 2#%!

~~Rehc:~~ ☹

~~Wy5vy:~~ ☹

~~Srvjy:~~ ☹

~~Whnl:~~ ☹

~~Rjc:~~ ☹

~~Dtwxg:~~ ☹

~~Gqau srube qb enuie:~~ ☹

(~~After~~ → ~~June 6/7, 2000)~~

(~~Read:~~ ☒ ~~No)~~

(~~Write:~~ ☒ ~~No)~~

(~~Speak:~~ ☒ ~~No)~~

(~~Walk:~~ ☒ ~~No)~~

(~~Run:~~ ☒ ~~No)~~

(~~Drive:~~ ☒ ~~No)~~

(~~Good sense of humor:~~ ☒ ~~No)~~

Now:

Read: ☑ Yes

Write: ☑ Yes

Speak: ☑ Yes

Walk: ☑ Yes

Run: ☒ No (yet)

Drive: ☑ Yes

Good sense of humor: ☑ Yes?

I'm truly, TRULY grateful to All of you! All of my family, all of my friends, the doctors, nurses, speech people, physical therapists, occupational therapists, all of the stroke survivors, emergency room people, S.F. Prosthetic Orthotic Service, optometrists, Apex Driving School, and so many other people, *AND* the Lord.

If I didn't mention you by name in this book, I'm so sorry! You deserve to be included too, so . . .

_____

(Write your name right above.)   ;)

THE END.

Wait! One more thing . . .

Maureen Twomey
San Francisco, CA (U.S.A.)

;-)

WRITING EXPERIENCE
Writer, San Francisco
A really good (great?) writer

Rtrebsertgh Ekibedht???@#%!!!
(Rehabilitation Expert, S.F.)
(CPMC Hospital, 6/6/2000 – 7/21/2000)
(Davies Campus, In-patient, 7/21/2000 –
9/14/2000)
(Davies Campus, Out-patient, 9/14/2000 –> ?)

Goldberg Moser O'Neill / Hill Holliday, S.F.
Copywriter (1/2000 – 6/2000 …)
Cisco Systems, NetAid, Audible.com, Micronpc.
com, inTune Hearing Center, HostPro, Web
Hosting, etc.

Freelancer; **Saatchi & Saatchi, Torrance**
Copywriter (11/1999 – 12/1999)
Toyota

TBWA\Chiat\Day, Venice/L.A.
Copywriter (6/1996 – 10/1999)
Nissan, Infiniti, The Weather Channel, ABC,
The Entertainment Ind. Foundation, New Business

MCA Records, Universal City

Editor and Chief Writer

AMP, MCA Records On Line (4/1996 – 6/1996)

Ketchum Advertising, Los Angeles

Copywriter (5/1994 – 4/1996)

Acura automobiles, PacifiCare, KFC Co-op, Aid
For AIDS New Business

OTHER EXPERIENCE
Ketchum Advertising, Los Angeles

Traffic Coordinator/Traffic Forwarder
(2/1993 – 5/1994)

Acura automobiles, American Lung Association

Bozell Advertising, Los Angeles

Account Group Assistant; Interoffice Coordinator
(10/1991 – 2/1993)

Rockwell International, Kawasaki Corp.,
Childhelp U.S.A.

**Rubin Postaer & Associates,
Los Angeles**

Account Group Assistant (11/1990 – 9/1991)

Honda automobiles

EDUCATION
June 6 and 7, 2000

I had to learn how to do it ALL over again: read,
write, speek, walk—and basically everything else.

WSAAA (Carson Roberts)
Creative Course
November 1994 – April 1995

The Bookshop
January – November 1992

University of California, Los Angeles
B.A. Communication Studies – June 1990

AWARDS AND HONORS

- 2015 Published my book, *Before, Afdre, and After*
- 1998 Clios (finalist)
- 1997 *Communiation Arts* Advertising Annual
- 1997 New York Art Directors (finalist)
- 1997 and 1996 Beldings
- 1997 One Show (Well, not yet a pencil; they displayed my work in their *Cross Dressing: The Role of Design in Advertising* exhibit, which is even more of an honor considering I'm not a transvestite)
- 1995 Best of Ketchum
- 1975 Published my book, *Sally the Snow Girl*

THE END.

REALLY

;)

Important Stuff

American Stroke Association

www.strokeassociation.org

National Stroke Association

www.stroke.org/site/PageNavigator/HOME

www.stroke.org/site/PageServer?pagename=FMD

California Pacific Medical Center (Sutter Health)

www.cpmc.org

www.cpmc.org/stroke

Davies Campus, California Pacific Medical Center (Sutter Health again)

www.cpmc.org/sift/?cid=11&si=cpmc&sw=0&st=davies%20 campus

The Critical Communicator

www.alimed.com/the-critical-communicator.html

The San Francisco Prosthetic Orthotic Service (S.F. POS)

http://sfpos.com

Daily Communicator

www.alimed.com/daily-communicator.html

Here's a link to many other interactive therapeutic things:

www.alimed.com/interactive-therapeutics/default.aspx

Ellen Gilbert, M.S., Speech-Language Pathologist

Specific Language / Learning Disability Specialty
(She recently retired from teaching.)

John Adams Center

www.ccsf.edu/en/our-campuses/john-adams2.html

CoWriter and Write:OutLoud

http://donjohnston.com/writing
http://donjohnston.com/writeoutloud

Stroke Survivors Starting Over, Peer Visitor Program

http://www.strokeassociation.org/STROKEORG/
Also search: Finding Support You Are Not Alone;
Stroke, Find a Support Group Peer Visitor Program

St. Mary's Medical Center

www.st-marys.org

Franklin, a Language Master

www.franklin.com

Dr. Iole Taddei, eye specialist

www.optometrists.org/Marin/index.html

Inspiration

www.inspiration.com/Inspiration

Apex Driving School, San Francisco

www.apexdrivingschool.com

Functional Solutions

www.BeAbleToDo.com

American Heart Association, Heart Walk

www.heartwalk.org/site/c.flKUIeOUIgJ8H/b.8939141/k.
BD45/Home.htm

Warner Coaching

http://warnercoaching.com

Other important names in this book:

Marc Deschenes and Laurie Brandalise (my headhunters)
John O'Dell, *Los Angeles Times*
Google maps
BATS Improv (http://www.improv.org)
Anne Lamott
E.L. Doctorow
AVON Walk for Breast Cancer (http://www.avonwalk.org)
inTune Hearing Center

Rick Steves' Europe (http://www.ricksteves.com)

COBRA

Apple (www.apple.com, not a real apple)

Microsoft Window (windows.microsoft.com/en-us/windows/
home)

Jenn Muranaka-Chaney, Art Director

Maureen Twomey, Copywriter ;)

Greg Behrendt

Sean Penn, Actor

Google and Bing

President Barack Obama

Facebook

U2

John McCain

Mitt Romney

Amazon.com (http://www.amazon.com)

eBay (http://www.ebay.com)

Mollie Caselli

And MOST Important:

Laura Mazer

Brooke Warner

Warner Coaching

Krissa Lagos, Copy Editor

Tabitha Lahr, Designer

And all my family and friends (again)

About the Author

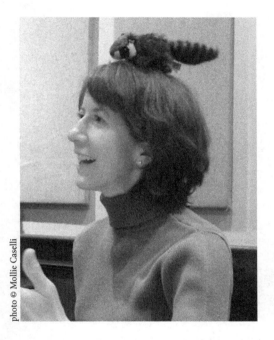

California native Maureen Twomey is
a writer. After graduating from UCLA
in 1990, she went on to work for
several advertising agencies, including
TBWA\Chiat\Day and Ketchum. She
now lives in San Francisco, where
she writes about her experience as a
survivor of a stroke.